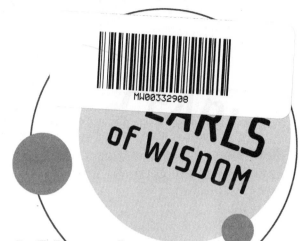

Medical-Surgical Nursing
Certification Examination
REVIEW

Editors

Scott H. Plantz, MD, FAAEM
Associate Professor, Chicago Medical School, Chicago, Illinois

E. John Wipfler III, MD, FACEP
Clinical Associate Professor of Surgery
University of Illinois College of Medicine
OSF Saint Francis Medical Center, Peoria, Illinois

Kelly Jo Cone, RN, PhD
Associate Professor, Graduate Program
OSF Saint Francis Medical Center College of Nursing, Peoria, Illinois

Sue Behrens, RN, MSN
Manager Trauma Services, OSF Saint Francis Medical Center, Peoria, Illinois

Colleen S. Ragon, RN, BSN
Life Flight, OSF Saint Francis Medical Center, Peoria, Illinois

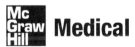 **Medical**

New York Chicago San Francisco Lisbon London Madrid Mexico City Milan
New Delhi San Juan Seoul Singapore Sydney Toronto

Medical Surgical Nursing Examination: Pearls of Wisdom

2 3 4 5 6 7 8 9 0   QPD/QPD   0 9 8 7

ISBN-13: 978-0-07-147040-7
ISBN-10: 0-07-147040-9

Notice

Medicine is an ever-changing science. As new research and clinical experience broaden our knowledge, changes in treatment and drug therapy are required. The authors and the publisher of this work have checked with sources believed to be reliable in their efforts to provide information that is complete and generally in accord with the standards accepted at the time of publication. However, in view of the possibility of human error or changes in medical sciences, neither the authors nor the publisher nor any other party who has been involved in the preparation or publication of this work warrants that the information contained herein is in every respect accurate or complete, and they disclaim all responsibility for any errors or omissions or for the results obtained from use of the information contained in this work. Readers are encouraged to confirm the information contained herein with other sources. For example and in particular, readers are advised to check the product information sheet included in the package of each drug they plan to administer to be certain that the information contained in this work is accurate and that changes have not been made in the recommended dose or in the contraindications for administration. This recommendation is of particular importance in connection with new or infrequently used drugs.

This book was set in Adobe Garamond by Aptara Inc.
The editors were Quincy McDonald and Christie Naglieri.
The production supervisor was Phil Galea.
Production management was provided by Aptara Inc.
The cover designer was Handel Low.
The text designer was Eve Siegel.
Quebecor Dubuque was printer and binder.

This book is printed on acid-free paper.

Library of Congress Cataloging-in-Publication Data

Medical-surgical nursing certification examination / Scott H. Plantz . . .
    [et al.].—1st ed.
        p. ; cm. – (Pearls of wisdom)
    Includes bibliographical references and index.
    ISBN-13: 978-0-07-147040-7 (pbk. : alk. paper)
    ISBN-10: 0-07-147040-9 (pbk. : alk. paper)
    1. Nursing–Examinations, questions, etc.   2. Operating room nursing–Examinations, questions, etc.
I. Plantz, Scott H.   II. Series.
    [DNLM: 1. Nursing Care–Examination Questions.   2. Perioperative Nursing–Examination Questions.
WY 18.2 M4893 2007]
RT55.M43 2007
610.73076—dc22
                                                    2006039220

DEDICATION

For the nursing staff at OSF Saint Francis Hospital . . . we hope you find this book a
great help in passing the medical-surgical exam!

Kelly Jo Cone, RN, PhD
Sue Behrens, RN, BSN
Colleen S. Ragon, RN, BSN

To my beautiful and supportive wife Diane, to my sister Jackie, who is one of the best nurses
in the world, to my wonderful parents Shirley (nurse) and Jack (surgeon), who have cared
for others all their lives, to my children Kate, Maria, Mathew, Laura, Rebecca, and Libby, and to
the excellent nursing staff at OSF Saint Francis Medical Center in Peoria, Illinois . . .
thank you for making this world a better place.

E. John Wipfler, III, MD, FACEP

To the nursing staff of Longview Regional Hospital in Longview, Texas and the nursing
staff of St. Anthony's Hospital, St. Petersburg, Florida—
Thank you for making my job enjoyable!

Scott H. Plantz, MD, FAAEM

CONTRIBUTING AUTHORS

William G. Gossman, MD
Associate Professor, St. Joe's Hospital
Creighton University, Omaha, Nebraska

Sheryl L. Gossman, RN, BSN
Project Director, Pearlsreview, Inc., Naperville, Illinois

Jacqueline Krajecki, RN, BSN
Registered Nurse, Sacred Heart Hospital
Pensacola, Florida

Nicholas Lorenzo, MD
Medical Director, Pearlsreview, Inc.
Omaha, Nebraska

Theresa Miller, RN, MSN, MHSA
Instructor, OSF Saint Francis Medical Center College of Nursing
Peoria, Illinois

TABLE OF CONTENTS

INTRODUCTION

Congratulations! The commitment to pursue certification reflects professionalism and a desire to demonstrate that you have obtained the knowledge required to be a skilled and competent medical-surgical nurse. This book is a good step toward that process. *Medical-Surgical* Certificiation Examination: Pearls of Wisdom has been designed to help you improve your performance on the Certified Medical-Surgical Nurse examination as well as help you identify some weak areas in your nursing knowledge. The format of this book is different than most of the common preparation review books in that you are not asked to select the best answer. Instead, the answer is provided for you. We have found that this method of exam review will give you the basic concepts necessary for passing the medical-surgical examination. Now a few words about the exam and its format, the intent of this book, and how this book is best utilized.

To be eligible for the medical-surgical examination, you must have a current registered nursing license without restrictions, suspension, probation, or any order arising from a nursing license authority that limits a nurse's ability to function in a hospital setting and perform those tasks normally associated with hospital nursing practice. If there is a current stipulation or action against a candidate's nursing license, but the candidate is permitted to perform all nursing functions, the candidate may be eligible to take the exam. Along with the above, you must have 2 years' experience in nursing practice and be a current member of the Medical-Surgical Nursing Association.

The format of the exam and its administration has changed during the past few years. It is now a computerized adaptive test (CAT), which means that the exam is adapted to your knowledge, skill, and ability level. You will take the exam alone at a computer station at an approved testing site. Each person's exam is unique in that the computer selects the questions based on your previous answer. For example, the computer will begin with an easy question. If you answer correctly, a question of greater or equal difficulty will be selected next. As you progress through the exam, the computer automatically calculates your skill level in each area of nursing knowledge. For those with "computer phobia," there is no need to worry. All keys on the keyboard will be inactive except for the space bar and the return key. They will be the only keys used. Practice questions will be given before the exam begins to acclimate you to the computer. However, during the exam, you will not be able to change an answer, skip questions, or return to a previous question.

The test ends when one of these three variables has been fulfilled: (1) the computer has determined that you are within the minimum competency level to pass, (2) you have answered 150 questions, or (3) you have reached the maximum time of 3 hours to complete the exam. A minimum of 100 questions must be answered before the computer will determine your competency level and there is no minimum time limit per question. Once the exam is completed, you will receive a pass/fail notification, but no numerical score will be assigned.

The exam covers the following practice areas:

Cardiovascular
Gastrointestional
Reproductive
Genitourinary and gynecologic
Eye, ears, nose, throat
Neurologic
Musculoskeletal, orthopedic, and trauma
Wounds
Infectious disease and immunology
Respiratory
Shock and resuscitation
Skin disorders
Endocrine
Patient care management
Patient education
Foundations of nursing
Legal and ethical nursing
Principles of medical-surgical nursing
Disruptions in homeostasis

So, how can this book help you prepare for this exam? *Medical-Surgical Nursing Certification Examination* is intended to serve as a study aid to improve performance on the exam. To achieve this goal, the text is divided into the major areas of emergency nursing study outlined above. Incorporated into these areas are the aspects that are covered on the Medical-Surgical exam. The questions are written in a straight-forward question/answer format and no intention has been made to mislead or "trick" the candidate.

The answer provided will be the best possible answer for that question. Unlike the Medical-Surgical exam, in which the answers given to a question may describe four different situations and you are to pick the *best*, this book looks at the underlying theory or idea behind the answer. For example, if a question is asked to determine the candidate's knowledge of the ABC's of resuscitation, the Medical-Surgical exam will list four actions that could be undertaken, all of which would be appropriate within the care of an unconscious patient. However, in determining which action should be taken first, the candidate should understand the principles of the ABCs of resuscitation and choose an answer related to determining and maintaining the airway. It is our intent that if the candidate understands the premise behind the answer, any list of situations can be asked, but the candidate will understand which situation is in line with the correct nursing theory. Therefore, this book should be an invaluable aid in determining your basic knowledge of nursing theories and medical facts.

In order to use this book to the fullest potential, the candidate should go through each question using a 3 × 5 card to cover the answer first in order to test his/her own knowledge. If upon reading the answer you do not understand the premise behind the answer, LOOK IT UP! Information that you will learn in response to seeking the answer will be more effectively retained than merely memorizing the correct answer without understanding the rationale behind it. A hollow bullet has been provided for your convenience to check off previously missed or answered questions, whichever is your preference.

Medical-Surgical Nursing Certification Examination is an interactive book designed to be used many times over. Test your knowledge by going through the book more that once and learn from your mistakes. Using this book in a group setting may also be helpful. Each individual in the group could determine their answer and then as a group compare. If there are discrepancies, look up the answer and determine why the answer is correct or incorrect.

Great care has been taken to determine the best possible questions and answers needed to pass the Medical-Surgical exam. Some questions and answers may seem outdated; however, we have attempted to form the questions so they are an accurate representation of those found on the Medical-Surgical exam. As always, we welcome your comments regarding questions, content, and any improvements or suggestions.

Study hard and good luck!

KC, SB, CR, EJW, and SP

Please email comments to: scotthuntlyplantz@yahoo.com

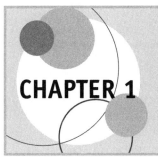

CHAPTER 1 Cardiovascular Pearls

○ **What is the leading cause of death and disease in the United States?**

Coronary artery disease (CAD), where arteries narrow from placques which partially or totally occlude the coronary artery vasculature.

○ **What is the usual cause of an AMI (acute myocardial infarction)?**

The coronary arteries develop a thrombus or blood clot formation at the site of a ruptured or narrow placque which leads to acute symptoms of chest pain (angina), hypotension, and dysfunction of the heart. Treatment is directed at reopening the artery and medical or surgical stabilization.

○ **What are the risk factors for coronary artery disease that cannot be modified?**

Gender (males higher risk), family history of heart disease, and increasing age.

○ **A medsurg nurse is discharging a patient who was diagnosed and treated for a heart attack. What are the risk factors for coronary artery disease than CAN be modified or treated to decrease this disease?**

Diet (lower fat, salt), hypertension, obesity, diabetes, cigarette smoking, sedentary lifestyle, high levels of triglycerides and low-density lipoprotein, and stress level (type A personality carries higher risks).

○ **What is the number one cause of preventable death in the United States?**

Cigarette smoking. A medsurg nurse, who convinces or assists their patients to stop smoking, does a tremendous service for the patient and their family.

○ **What is the *most common* symptom of aortic dissection?**

Interscapular back pain. Classically is a sharp, tearing, severe pain.

○ **What side effect is expected with too rapid an infusion of procainamide?**

Hypotension. Other side effects include: myocardial depression, QRS/QT prolongation, V-fib, and torsade de pointes.

○ **What are the adverse drug effects of lidocaine?**

Drowsiness, nausea, vertigo, confusion, ataxia, tinnitus, muscle twitching, respiratory depression, and psychosis. ECG changes may be seen also.

O   **When is dobutamine used in CHF?**

Potent inotrope with some vasodilation activity, used when heart failure is not accompanied by severe hypotension. Dobutamine decreases afterload and increases contractility.

O   **When is dopamine selected in CHF?**

Vasoconstrictor and positive inotrope, is used to increase cardiac output, especially if shock is present.

O   **Key questions a medsurg nurse should ask patients regarding family history of cardiovascular disorders?**

Hypertension, coronary artery disease, vascular disease, sudden death (arrhythmia), or hyperlipidemia.

O   **What is sinus tachycardia?**

Heart rate greater than 100 beats per minute and every QRS complex follows a P wave.

O   **What is sinus bradycardia?**

Heart rate less than 60 beats per minute and every QRS complex follows a P wave.

O   **How is atrial flutter treated?**

Initiate A-V nodal blockade with β-adrenergic or calcium channel blockers or with digoxin. If necessary, in a stable patient, attempt chemical cardioversion with a class IA agent such as procainamide or quinidine after digitalization. If such treatment fails, or if patient is unstable and requires immediate electrocardioversion, do so with 25–50 J. Sedation should be considered prior to electrical cardioversion.

O   **What are the causes of atrial fibrillation?**

Hypertension, rheumatic heart disease, pneumonia, thyrotoxicosis, and ischemic heart disease are common causes. Pericarditis, ETOH intoxication, PE, CHF, and COPD are other causes.

O   **How is atrial fibrillation treated?**

If patient is stable then control a fast ventricular rate with diltiazem bolus and/or IV infusion; consider digitalis, and if indicated, convert with procainamide, quinidine, or verapamil. Synchronized cardioversion at 100–200 J in an unstable patient requiring cardioversion. In a stable patient with a-fib of unclear duration, anticoagulation for 2–3 weeks should be considered prior to chemical or electrical cardioversion in order to decrease the chance of an embolic stroke or other embolic problem.

O   **What are some causes of SVT (supraventricular tachycardia)?**

SVT may be due to digitalis toxicity (25% of digitalis induced arrhythmias), pericarditis, MI, COPD, preexcitation syndromes, mitral valve prolapse, rheumatic heart disease, pneumonia, drug and alcohol abuse.

O   **Describe the key features of Mobitz I (Wenckebach) 2° AV block.**

Progressive prolongation of the PR interval over several heartbeats seen on the ECG or telemetry trip until atrial impulse is not conducted, resulting in a skipped beat (QRS complex), then the sequence repeats itself. If symptomatic, atropine, and possibly transcutaneous/transvenous pacing are indicated.

O   **Describe the features and treatment of Mobitz II 2° AV block.**

Constant PR interval. One or more beats fail to conduct interspersed with normally conducted P-waves. More serious than Mobitz I. Treat with atropine and consider transcutaneous/transvenous pacing.

○ **Name five causes of mesenteric ischemia.**

Arterial thrombosis at sites of atherosclerotic plaques, emboli from left atrium in patients with a-fib or rheumatic heart disease who are not anticoagulated, arterial embolism most common to the superior mesenteric artery, insufficient arterial flow, and venous thrombosis.

○ **What is the *most common* source for acute mesenteric ischemia.**

Arterial embolism 40–50%. Source is usually the heart, most often from a mural thrombus (recent MI often). Most common point of obstruction is the superior mesenteric artery.

○ **What is Buerger's disease?**

Buerger's disease is also called thromboangiitis obliterans, an inflammatory, nonatheromatous occlusive condition that causes segmental lesions and thrombus formation in medium and small arteries with less blood flow to the feet and legs, usually in heavy smokers, males in their 20s and 30s; symptoms are usually claudication, pain, cold feet, eventual redness or cyanosis of legs, may lead to gangrene and amputation.

○ **What are contraindications to β-blockers?**

CHF, variant angina, AV block, COPD, asthma (relative), bradycardia, hypotension, and insulin dependent diabetes mellitus (IDDM). Also, patients with recent cocaine use should not receive β-blockers.

○ **What are the three types of angina?**

Stable, unstable (has increased in frequency, duration, severity, or quality and occurs with minimal exertion and rest), and Prinzmetal's or variant (angina that occurs at rest or during sleep, long after exercise).

○ **A patient who is day 1 after an acute myocardial infarction (AMI), develops a new loud (4/6) systolic murmur along the left sternal border and pulmonary edema. Diagnosis?**

Ventricular septal rupture. Diagnosis is confirmed with Swan-Ganz catheterization or echo. Treatment includes nitroprusside for afterload reduction and possible intra-aortic balloon pump followed by surgical repair.

○ **In a patient who has recently suffered an AMI, when would cardiac rupture be expected?**

In the first 5 days, post-MI 50% of all ruptures occur, while 90% occur within the first 14 days post MI.

○ **A patient is readmitted to the floor 2 weeks post AMI with chest pain, fever, and pleuropericarditis. A pleural effusion is seen on CXR. Diagnosis?**

Dressler's (postmyocardial infarction) syndrome which is caused by an immunologic reaction to myocardial antigens.

○ **Can patients be retreated with streptokinase or APSAC?**

No, because antibodies persist for 6 months.

○ **What is the *most common* symptom of acute pericarditis?**

Sharp or stabbing retrosternal or precordial chest pain, and the pain increases when supine and decreases when sitting-up and leaning forward. Pain may be increased with movement and deep breaths. Other symptoms include fever, dyspnea described as pain with inspiration, and dysphagia.

○ **What physical findings are associated with acute pericarditis?**

Pericardial friction rub is the most common. Rub is best heard at the left sternal border or apex in a sitting leaning forward position. Other findings include fever and tachycardia.

○ **What are the *most common* symptoms and signs of PE (pulmonary embolus)?**

Tachypnea (92%)
Chest Pain (88%)
Dyspnea (84%)
Anxiety (59%)
Tachycardia (44%)
Fever (43%)
DVT (32%)
Hypotension (25%).
Syncope (13%)

○ **What is the *most common* cause of mitral stenosis?**

Rheumatic heart disease. The most common initial symptom is dyspnea.

○ **What are the *most common* causes of acute mitral regurgitation?**

Rupture of the chordae tendineae, rupture of the papillary muscles, or perforation of the valve leaflets. Common causes include AMI and infectious endocarditis.

○ **What are the two *most common* causes of valvular aortic stenosis?**

Rheumatic heart disease and congenital bicuspid valve.

○ **What triad of symptoms is characteristic of aortic stenosis?**

Syncope, angina, and left heart failure. As the disease progresses, systolic BP decreases and pulse pressure narrows.

○ **What are the signs and symptoms of *acute* aortic regurgitation?**

Dyspnea, tachycardia, tachypnea, and chest pain. Causes include: infectious endocarditis, acute rheumatic fever, trauma, spontaneous rupture of valve leaflets, or aortic dissection.

○ **What physical findings are characteristic of *chronic* aortic regurgitation?**

Bobbing of the head with systole, bounding carotid pulse (water-hammer), pistol shot sound, the to-and-fro murmur of Duroziez's sign over the femoral arteries, and capillary pulsation of the nailbeds (Quincke's sign).

○ **What is the *most common* cause of tricuspid stenosis?**

Rheumatic heart disease.

○ **What are the two conditions that significantly increase the risk for endocarditis?**

Having a damaged heart valve (congenital heart or heart valve disease, rheumatic fever, etc.) or having a prosthetic heart valve.

○   **What is the classic physical sign of endocarditis?**

A loud regurgitant heart murmur or a murmur that has changed in intensity or type.

○   **What are Janeway lesions?**

Purple-colored circular flat rashes (macules) on the palms or soles, due to embolic pieces of clot and infected thrombi that break free of endocarditis and float to the distal circulation in the feet and hands. Other signs include petechiae of the skin and mucous membranes and splinter hemorrhages under the nails.

○   **What can a medsurg nurse do to help prevent endocarditis?**

Help screen for and identify patients at risk for endocarditis, such as those with heart valve disease or prosthetic heart valves who are undergoing invasive procedures such as surgery of the GI or GU tract, gynecologic procedures, childbirth, or dental work. Prophylactic antibiotic administration may be indicated depending upon the risks involved and likelihood of bacteremia with subsequent endocarditis.

○   **Define a hypertensive emergency.**

Increased BP with associated end-organ dysfunction or damage. A controlled drop in BP over 1 hour should be attempted.

○   **Define a hypertensive urgency.**

BP elevated to dangerous level, typically a diastolic greater than 115 mm Hg. Gradually reduce BP over 24–48 hours.

○   **Define uncomplicated hypertension.**

Diastolic BP more than 90 but less than 115 mm Hg with no symptoms of end-organ damage. Does not require acute treatment, but further management and testing is indicated.

○   **What lab findings would suggest a hypertensive emergency?**

UA—RBCs, red cell casts, and proteinuria.
BUN and CR—elevated (renal impairment).
X-ray—Aortic dissection, pulmonary edema, or coarctation of the aorta.
ECG—Left ventricular hypertrophy and cardiac ischemia.

○   **In general, how quickly should severe elevations in BP (>210/130) be treated?**

Use medications to decrease the diastolic blood pressure 20–30% over 30–60 minutes.

○   **What drugs should be used to lower BP in a patient with thoracic aortic dissection?**

Sodium nitroprusside, propranolol, or labetalol. An arterial line should be considered to closely monitor the blood pressure.

○   **What drug can be used for all hypertensive emergencies?**

Sodium nitroprusside (not DOC for eclampsia). Sodium nitroprusside works through production of cGMP which relaxes smooth muscle. This results in decreased preload and afterload, decreased oxygen demand, slight increased heart rate with no change in myocardial blood flow, cardiac output, or renal blood flow. Duration of action is 1–2 minutes. Sometimes, ß-blockade is required to treat rebound tachycardia.

○ **What is the *most common* complication of nitroprusside?**

Hypotension. Thiocyanate toxicity with blurred vision, tinnitus, change in mental status, muscle weakness, and seizures is seen more often in patients with renal failure and after prolonged infusions. Cyanide toxicity is uncommon, it may occur with hepatic dysfunction, after prolonged infusions, and in rates greater than 10 µg/kg per minute.

○ **A patient presents with sudden onset of chest pain and back pain. Further work-up reveals an ischemic right leg. Diagnosis?**

Suspect an acute aortic dissection when chest or back pain is associated with ischemic or neurologic defects. The dissection progresses and causes occlusion of aortic vasculature such as the iliac or femoral artery resulting in loss of flow and pulse.

○ **What physical findings are suspicious for acute aortic dissection?**

BP differences between arms, cardiac tamponade, and aortic insufficiency murmur.
An abnormal ECG may also be present.

○ **In a patient with an abdominal mass and a suspected ruptured AAA, what x-ray study should be ordered?**

None. They should go to the OR ASAP if fairly certain of the diagnosis. About 60% of AAAs will have "eggshell" calcifications and thus appear on lateral abdominal x-ray. If time allows, then a bedside ultrasound is 98% diagnostic of AAA but limited ability to detect leakage. Abdominal CT scan is most accurate and assists the surgeon in identifying optimum treatment.

○ **A cyanotic patient has a low oxygen saturation measured on ABG. What type of cyanosis does this patient have?**

Central.

○ **What is peripheral cyanosis?**

When the patient has blue or dark colored extremities but the ABG reveals oxygen saturation within normal; in these cases shunting or increased O_2 extraction is taking place.

○ **Name the two primary causes (groups) of peripheral cyanosis.**

Cyanosis with a normal SaO_2 can be due to:
decreased cardiac output.
 redistribution—may be 2° to shock, DIC, hypothermia, vascular obstruction.

○ **Name the causes of central cyanosis.**

The causes of cyanosis with a decreased SaO_2 are:
decreased PaO_2, or decreased O_2 diffusion.
hypoventilation.

V-Q mismatch, pulmonary shunting.

dysfunctional hemoglobin (includes sickle cell crisis, drug-induced hemoglobinopathies).

Note: Hb-CO (carbon monoxide poisoning) does not cause cyanosis (though the cherry red appearance of skin and mucous membranes could suggest a cyanosis).

○ **What is the *most common* conduction disturbance in acute myocardial infarction?**

First-degree AV block.

○ **What is the treatment for torsade de pointes?**

Treatment includes techniques to accelerate the heart rate, shortening the duration of ventricular repolarization. This may be accomplished with isoproterenol IV infusion (target heart rate of 90), temporary pacing, or with magnesium sulfate. If indicated then defibrillation should be done. Any precipitating agent should be discontinued. Drugs which increase or prolong repolarization, and therefore exacerbate torsade de pointes, include Class IA antiarrhythmics (quinidine, procainamide, disopyramide), tricyclic antidepressants, phenothiazines, and others causes.

○ **Dobutamine in moderate doses causes what cardiovascular effects?**

Decreased peripheral vascular resistance and pulmonary occlusive pressure, and positive inotropic stimulation of the heart.

○ **What is the best treatment for an unstable patient with Wolff-Parkinson-White syndrome presenting with rapid atrial fibrillation?**

Synchronized cardioversion 50–100 J. Sedation should always be considered prior.

○ **What is the best treatment for a verapamil-induced bradycardia?**

Calcium chloride 10%, give 10–20 ml IV. (This is about 10–20 mg/kg, use 10–30 mg/kg in children.) CaCl should be given via a central line or PIC line if possible due to severe tissue damage that may occur with accidental subcutaneous infiltration. If a peripheral line is used, most sources recommend calcium gluconate rather than the potentially harmful calcium chloride.

○ **What are the signs and symptoms of acute pericardial tamponade?**

Triad of hypotension, elevated CVP, and tachycardia is usually indicative of either acute pericardial tamponade or a tension pneumothorax in a traumatized patient. Muffled heart tones may be auscultated. Echocardiography is urgently needed to differentiate and diagnosis.

○ **What EKG finding is pathognomonic of pericardial tamponade?**

Total electrical alternans. Pulsus paradoxus is nonspecific. Muffled heart tones are subjective findings and are difficult to appreciate.

○ **What is the *most common* site of thrombophlebitis?**

The deep muscles of the calves, particularly the soleus muscle.

○ **What is the *most common* cause of acute aortic regurgitation?**

Infectious endocarditis.

○ **What are the two *most common* causes of pulsus paradoxus?**

COPD and asthma.

○ **What does Beck's triad consist of?**

Hypotension, elevated CVP (distended neck veins), and distant muffled heart sounds.

○ **What does the presence of Beck's triad indicate?**

Acute pericardial tamponade.

○ **What is the *most common* symptom in leaking or expanding abdominal aortic aneurysms?**

Pain, typically in the midabdomen or back, and when it expands it may cause severe tearing flank pain (bilateral or unilateral simulating a kidney stone).

○ **What is the *most common* dysrhythmia associated with Wolff-Parkinson-White syndrome?**

Paroxysmal atrial tachycardia.

○ **What are the symptoms and signs of aortic stenosis?**

Exertional dyspnea, angina, and syncope.
Narrowed pulse pressure with decreased SBP.
Slow carotid upstroke.
Prominent S_4.

○ **What drugs are contraindicated for treatment of torsade de pointes?**

A drug which prolongs repolarization (QT interval). For example, class Ia antiarrhythmics (quinidine, procainamide).
Other drugs that share this effect include TCAs, disopyramide, and phenothiazines.

○ **What is the treatment of torsade de pointes?**

Pacemaker cranked to 90–120 bpm to "overdrive" pace.
Isoproterenol.
Magnesium sulfate 2 g IV.

The goal is to accelerate the heart rate and shorten ventricular repolarization.

○ **What drugs are commonly associated with torsade de pointes?**

Type I-A antiarrhythmics—quinidine and procainamide.
These drugs lengthen the Q-T interval.

○ **What is the *most common* cause of multifocal atrial tachycardia?**

COPD.

○ **What is the treatment for multifocal atrial tachycardia?**

Treat underlying disorder.

Magnesium sulfate 2 g over 60 seconds (with supplemental potassium to maintain serum K^+ above 4 mEq/l).

○ **What is the treatment of ectopic SVT due to digitalis toxicity?**

Stop digitalis, correct hypokalemia, consider digoxin-specific antibody fragments (Fab), magnesium IV, lidocaine IV or phenytoin IV.

○ **What is the treatment for verapamil-induced hypotension?**

Calcium gluconate 1 g IV over several minutes.

○ **What are the three types of cardiomyopathy and which type is *most common*?**

Dilated or congestive (most common), hypertrophic (hypertrophied left ventricle is small, unable to relax and fill properly), and restrictive cardiomyopathy (rare; stiff ventricles).

○ **What are the causes of dilated cardiomyopathy?**

Infection, metabolic and immunologic disorders, chronic alcohol abuse, pregnancy and postpartum disorders, and coronary artery disease.

○ **What is the number one cause of right-sided heart failure?**

Left-sided heart failure (from AMI, VSD, cardiomyopathy, constrictive pericarditis, increased circulating blood volume, aortic and mitral valve stenosis or insufficiency, and other causes).

○ **What are causes of high-output heart failure?**

Thyrotoxicosis, anemia, pregnancy, beriberi, and arteriovenous fistula

○ **What are the treatment options for digitalis toxicity.**

Oral activated charcoal. Consider charcoal with sorbital if acute overdose.

Phenytoin (Dilantin) for ventricular arrhythmias (it increases AV node conduction) or lidocaine.

Atropine or pace for bradyarrthymias.

Digoxin specific Fab (Digibind) is expensive but very effective.

○ **What is the drug of choice for digitalis toxicity resulting in a ventricular arrhythmia?**

Phenytoin and digoxin specific Fab (Dilantin and Digibind).

○ **What traditional antiarrhythmic agents may be used to treat digitalis induced ventricular arrhythmias in addition to phenytoin?**

Lidocaine and bretylium. Procainamide and quinidine are contraindicated in digitalis toxicity.

○ **What effect do β-blockers have on Prinzmetal's variant angina?**

β-blockers typically worsen the syndrome by allowing unopposed α–adrenergic stimulation of the coronary arteries.

○ **What common drugs cause bradycardia?**

Agents such as β-blockers, cardiac glycosides, pilocarpine, and cholinesterase inhibitors such as organophosphates are responsible for bradycardia.

○ **What common drugs cause tachycardia?**

Sympathomimetics such as amphetamines and cocaine, and anticholinergics, such as atropine and cyclic antidepressants, commonly cause tachycardia.

○ **What are the three types of mechanical disruption in patients with valvular heart disease?**

Prolapse of the valve (such as mitral valve prolapse), narrowing (stenosis) of the valve opening, or incomplete closure of the valve (insufficiency).

○ **What valvular lesion is most likely to cause syncope?**

Aortic stenosis.

○ **What is the *most common* valvular disorder in the United States?**

Mitral valve prolapse.

○ **What is an interesting diagnostic feature of aortic regurgitation?**

Head bobbing.

○ **What is the *most common* arrhythmia associated with digitalis?**

PVC (60%).
Ectopic SVT (25%).
AV block (20%).

○ **What is the *most common* arrhythmia in mitral stenosis?**

Atrial fibrillation due to atrial distention

○ **A medsurg nurse is administering coumadin (warfarin) to a patient with deep vein thrombophlebitis. What laboratory test is used to indicate coumadin is at therapeutic levels, and what is the ideal result?**

Prothrombin time (PT). When the patient's PT is 1 ½–2 times the control, or an INR of 2–3, then the blood is appropriately anticoagulated. The PTT is used to determine the therapeutic activity of heparin.

○ **The *most common* cause of CHF in an adult is:**

Hypertension.

○ **What is considered the cornerstone of drug therapy for patients with chronic congestive heart failure?**

An ACE inhibitor to decrease afterload combined with a β-blocker.

○ **What effect does the Valsalva's maneuver have on the heart?**

Valsalva decreases blood return to both the right and left ventricles. All murmurs decrease in intensity except IHSS.

○ **In asthmatic patient suddenly develops a supraventricular tachycardia. Blood pressure is normal and the QRS complex is also narrow. What therapy is most appropriate?**

Verapamil.

Avoid the use of adenosine as it is relatively contraindicated and may exacerbate bronchospasm in asthmatic patients. Also avoid β-blockers.

○ **In endocarditis (all comers), what is the most commonly involved cardiac valve?**

Mitral > Aortic > Tricuspid > Pulmonic.

○ **What is the most reliable site for detecting central cyanosis?**

The tongue.

○ **When do CK-MB levels first begin to rise and when do they peak in an MI?**

CK-MB earliest rise 6–8 hours.

Peak 24–30 hours.

Normalizes 48 hours.

○ **When does LDH first begin to rise and when does it peak in an MI?**

LDH-I (from heart) earliest rise 12–24 hours.

Peak 48 to 96 hours.

○ **When do troponin levels first begin to rise and when do they peak in an MI?**

Troponin rises as early as 6–12 hours.

Peak at 14 hours, and again several days later (biphasic peak).

○ **What is the effect of nitrates on preload and afterload?**

Nitrates mostly dilate veins and venules to decrease preload, but also decrease afterload.

○ *Inferior* **wall MIs commonly lead to what two types of heart block (via mechanism of damage to autonomic fibers in the atrial septum giving increased vagal tone impairing AV node conduction)?**

First-degree AV block.

Mobitz Type I (Wenckebach) second-degree AV block.

Sinus bradycardia can also occur.

Progression to complete AV block is *not* common.

○ *Anterior* **wall MIs may directly damage intracardiac conduction. This may lead to what type of arrhythmias?**

The *dangerous* type! Mobitz II second-degree AV block that can suddenly progress to complete AV block.

○ **What is the *most common* cause of acute aortic regurgitation?**

Infectious endocarditis.

○ **What is the *most common* congenital valvular disease?**

Bicuspid aortic valve.

○ **What infarct is most commonly associated with acute mitral regurgitation?**

Inferior wall.

○ **A patient is digitalis toxic. What electrolytes will need to be replaced?**

It is important to replace potassium and magnesium.

○ **What is the *most common* complication of verapamil and how should it be treated?**

Hypotension, which is treated with IV fluids and calcium gluconate IV over 2–3 minutes.

○ **What is a common pathologic cause of an S_3?**

Congestive heart failure.

○ **What is the pathologic cause of an S_4?**

Often decreased left ventricular compliance due to acute ischemia.
Other causes include: aortic stenosis, subaortic stenosis, HTN, coronary artery disease, myocardiopathy, anemia, and hyperthyroidism.

○ **Does furosemide affect preload or afterload?**

Furosemide decreases preload by causing initial vasodilation and later diuresis.

○ **What is the *most common* cause of tricuspid regurgitation?**

Right heart failure secondary to left heart failure, typically caused by mitral stenosis.

○ **What type of abnormal cardiac rhythm can be slowed through Valsalva maneuvers and/or carotid massage?**

Supraventricular rhythms.

○ **Name some common Valsalva maneuvers.**

Holding the breath, stimulation of the gag reflex, squatting, pressure on the eyeball, or immersing the face in ice water.

○ **80–90% of patients who experience sudden nontraumatic cardiac arrest are in what rhythm?**

Ventricular fibrillation. Early defibrillation is the key. In an acute MI, the infarction zone becomes electrically unstable. Ventricular fibrillation is most common during original coronary occlusion or when the coronaries begin to reperfuse.

○ **What is the *most common* cause of death within the first few hours following an MI?**

Cardiac dysrhythmias, generally V-fib.

○ **A client with a history of congestive heart failure presents with coarse rales, pink frothy sputum, restlessness, and dyspnea. What would you suspect is the cause?**

Pulmonary edema.

○ **What would be the best position for this client in bed?**

High Fowler's position (sitting upright).

○ **During the first hours after a myocardial infarction, why is it important to monitor the patient's ECG?**

Arrhythmias are the leading cause of death following an infarct.

○ **You auscultate an S₃ heart sound in a patient with CHF. What significance does this sound have?**

Probably a decreased ventricular wall compliance from a past infarction.

○ **A client's blood pressure is 150/90 with no previous history of hypertension. The patient asks if he will have to be put on medication. How should you respond?**

A one time elevated blood pressure reading does not indicate hypertension. The patient should have his blood pressure taken several more times (at least once a week × 3 weeks, in a relaxed setting) before a diagnosis can be made.

○ **A 49-year-old male is transferred from the coronary ICU to the medsurg floor on telemetry. He received streptokinase for his heart attack the day before. What is the most harmful complication of this medication that a medsurg nurse should assess for?**

Bleeding.

○ **To prevent a patient's nitroglycerin tablets from going stale and becoming ineffective, how often should they be replaced?**

Every 6 months. Nitroglycerin *spray* has a shelf life of up to 2 years.

○ **Why should you assess for digitalis toxicity when a patient is taking Lanoxin (digoxin) and lasix?**

Lasix decreases the serum potassium level which can increase the toxic effects of digitalis.

○ **What cardiac abnormality can occur with theophylline levels above 35 mcg/ml?**

Ventricular arrhythmias.

○ **What type of weather tends to aggravate angina pectoris?**

Cold weather.

○ **What environmental factors contribute the most to coronary artery disease?**

Diet.

○ **What important side effect of Inderal (propranolol hydrochloride) should you assess for?**

Slowed pulse rate and associated dyshythmias.

○ **What is the best position for a patient in acute CHF with a normal blood pressure, and why?**

High Fowler's. It decreases venous return and allows for maximum lung expansion. If the patient is hypotensive, then the head should be lowered to improve brain blood flow and to prevent stroke and mental status changes.

○ **How can you determine if the chest pain, a patient experiences, is due to angina or a myocardial infarction?**

It may be difficult. Anginal pain is usually relieved by resting, lying down, oxygen, and/or by administering nitroglycerin.

○ **What is the cause of pain in a myocardial infarction?**

Oxygen deprived ischemic cardiac muscle.

○ **When applying nitroglycerin paste, what should you avoid?**

Getting the paste on your own skin.

○ **What information does an EKG (ECG) provide?**

It reflects the electrical impulses transmitted through the heart and can be an indicator of the functional status of the heart muscle and contractile responses of the ventricles.

○ **Which coronary artery is associated with each of the following MI infarct areas diagnosed on an EKG (ECG): inferior MI, anterior MI, lateral MI?**

The infarct location is directly related to disease in a particular coronary artery:
An inferior MI correlates with disease in the right coronary artery, an anterior MI correlates with the left anterior descending artery (LAD), and a lateral MI correlates with disease in the circumflex coronary artery.

○ **What is the purpose of a cardiac catheterization?**

To assess the extent of coronary artery blockage.

○ **How can percutaneous transluminal coronary angioplasty cause a fluid volume deficit?**

The contrast medium used can act as an osmotic diuretic and diuresis can result.

○ **What vital sign should be monitored closely during administration of nitroglycerin?**

Blood pressure. The vasodilation can sometimes cause significant hypotension. Patients who receive NTG in the hospital should have an IV in place in case a fluid bolus is needed after NTG is given.

○ **What should be done if premature ventricular contractions (PVCs) at a rate of 8–10 per minute are noticed on a patient's monitor?**

Notify the physician. PVCs, which are new and greater that 5–6 per minute are considered dangerous in a patient with cardiac ischemia.

○ **How could a patient's pulse be described if atrial fibrillation is present?**

Irregular with a variable rate.

○ **What would be the purpose of administering digoxin (Lanoxin) intravenously to a patient with CHF?**

Lanoxin can help strengthen myocardial contractions and thus help increase cardiac output, which will help reduce pulmonary edema.

○ **What is the purpose of administering alteplase (tPA) during the first 6 hours following onset of chest pain in a myocardial infarction?**

It is able to lyse the clot that is blocking the coronary artery and help restore blood flow to the heart muscles and tissue.

○ **Why is there a potential for blood clot formation in a patient with atrial fibrillation?**

The ineffective contractions of the atria cause blood stasis and thus clot formation.

○ **According to the American Heart Association, what is the definition of hypertension?**

Consistent blood pressure readings of a systolic above 140 and a diastolic above 90, documented on two or more consecutive readings over a 2-week period.

○ **What are the four types of hypertension (HTN)?**

Primary (or essential HTN), which is hypertension of unknown cause;
Secondary (from known cause such as renovascular disease, coarctation of the aorta, etc.);
Accelerated (diastolic BP above 120 mm Hg and rapid vascular changes);
Malignant (diastolic BP above 140 mm HG)

○ **What is the primary effect of nitroglycerin?**

Peripheral vasodilatation, which reduces myocardial oxygen consumption and workload.

○ **What should a primary nursing assessment especially include during the administration of TPA?**

Signs and symptoms of spontaneous bleeding.

○ **A patient taking Lanoxin complains of anorexia, nausea, and vomiting. What should you suspect?**

Digitalis toxicity.

○ **What type of visual changes occur with digitalis toxicity?**

"Yellow-colored" vision and halos.

○ **What are the common side effects of nitroglycerin?**

Headache, hypotension, and dizziness.

○ **What is coronary percutaneous transluminal coronary angioplasty (PTCA)?**

A balloon tipped catheter is inserted into the coronary artery and compresses outward against the plaque in hopes of dilating the artery. A stent (metal or other material) is often used to keep the narrow artery open longer.

○ **When chest pain occurs, what is the time interval for administration of nitroglycerin tablets or spray?**

Immediate administration with subsequent doses at 5 minute intervals until the pain has resolved or a total of three tablets have been taken. Additional NTG tablets or spray may be given as long as the patient has chest pain and the blood pressure is satisfactory. One table of NTG is 400 μg. One spray of NTG is also 400 μg.

○ **A medsurg nurse is discharging a patient with newly diagnosed angina who received angioplasty. The nurse should tell the patient to do what, if his pain is unresolved after taking three nitroglycerin tablets?**

Seek medical treatment immediately.

○ **Where is the dorsalis pedis pulse palpated?**

Medial aspect of the dorsal surface of the foot.

○ **At what time is a patient at greatest risk of dying from an acute myocardial infarction (AMI)?**

The first 24–48 hours after an acute myocardial infarction. The 30-day death rate is 7% for hospitalized patients, and 14% for unhospitalized AMI victims.

○ **What does paroxysmal nocturnal dyspnea (PND) indicate?**

Congestive heart failure. Patients with this go to sleep feeling well, then while laying flat the lungs become congested and they awake with significant shortness of breath (dyspnea).

○ **What may hypotension indicate in a patient with an MI?**

Cardiogenic shock.

○ **How does nitroglycerine help relieve the pain associated with angina and an MI?**

It causes coronary artery vasodilatation leading to an increase in blood flow to the cardiac muscle.

○ **What does the term "silent myocardial infarction" indicate?**

An MI that produces no chest pain or other symptoms. This is more common in diabetics and the elderly.

○ **What are the adverse reactions to verapamil?**

Headaches, hypotension, atrial-ventricular conduction disturbances, dizziness, and hypotension.

○ **What is the treatment for mild to moderate varicose veins?**

Antiembolism stockings and moderate walking, which will minimize venous pooling.

○ **When administering a nitroprusside sodium IV, what special care should be taken with the medication bag?**

Wrap the IV bag in foil to shield it from light (light causes degradation of the drug)

○ **What are the alterable risk factors for coronary artery disease?**

High cholesterol and/or triglyceride levels, diabetes, hypertension, and cigarette smoking.

○ **What are the major complications of an acute myocardial infarction?**

Thromboembolism, cardiogenic shock, left ventricular rupture, acute heart failure, and arrhythmias.

○ **When assessing a patient's heart, where is the point of maximal impulse (PMI) usually found?**

Fifth intercostal space, left midclavicular line.

○ **What does ST elevation on a 12 lead ECG indicate?**

Injury to cardiac muscle. If noted in several leads then this patient may be having an AMI.

○ **Describe the classic diagnostic criteria for an acute Inferior Wall MI on a 12 lead ECG.**

ST elevation greater than 2 mm in contiguous leads II, III, and AVF.

○ **What is the medical criteria used to determine the need for an emergency thoracotomy?**

Penetration chest trauma, tension pneumothorax, and crush injuries to the chest.

○ **What is the common dysrhythmia associated with cardiac reperfusion after the administration of thrombolytics?**

Accelerated idioventricular rhythm.

○ **A patient in v-fib with no pulse has undergone attempted defibrillation with 360 J and v-fib remains on the monitor. What is the next step?**

Resume CPR, monitor patient closely for signs of revival, provide ACLS medications per protocol, and every 2 minutes defibrillate at 360 J if indicated. . . . .

○ **What drugs can be administered via endotracheal tube?**

NAVEL-Naloxone, Atropine, Valium, Epinephrine, and Lidocaine.

○ **The patient's tPA infusion is complete. What should the nurse do before disconnecting the infusion?**

Flush the line to ensure administration of all the drug.

○ **During tPA administration, you note a change in the patient's level of consciousness and weakness in the extremities. What serious complication of tPA administration should you suspect?**

Intracranial hemorrhage. This patient should go to CT scan immediately after stabilization.

○ **What should you consider in a patient who has no pulse, but a rhythm on the monitor?**

Hypovolemia, cardiac tamponade, tension pneumothorax, acidosis, pulmonary embolism, and hypoxemia are possible causes of PEA—pulseless electrical activity.

○ **What are the common conversion dysrhythmias seen with adenosine administration?**

Bradycardia, short periods of asystole, and heart block (briefly, rapidly resolves). Patients often will get a short 1–2 second episode of sharp chest pain also.

○ **A 60-year-old female presents with a swollen, red, lower left leg and a positive Homans' sign. What should you suspect?**

Deep vein thrombosis.

○ **A medsurg nurse has a patient with moderate congestive heart failure (CHF) who is having pain with breathing, and morphine is administered. What effect does morphine have on the patient in acute CHF?**

Reduces preload, reduces respiratory rate, and decreases anxiety.

○ **Why is it important from a psychological standpoint to control the chest pain of a client having a myocardial infarction?**

Pain causes the release of catecholamines, which cause increased heart rate and increased forceful contractions both of which create additional oxygen demands on the heart. Controlling pain should lessen oxygen demand of the heart.

○ **What is a priority nursing diagnosis for the client who has suffered a cardiac contusion?**

Risk for potential decreased cardiac output.

○ **What complications of a cardiac contusion should the nurse monitor the patient for?**

Dysrhythmias, pericardial tamponade, coronary artery occlusion, or valvular damage.

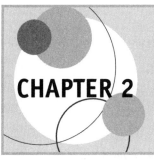

CHAPTER 2

Musculoskeletal, Trauma, and Orthopedic Pearls

○ **A 17-year-old male is admitted to the surgery floor with a gunshot wound to the chest and a chest tube. He has a cough with hemoptysis. Appropriate nursing PPE would include_____.**

Scene safety and staff safety, using personal protective equipment (PPE), universal precautions, and body substance isolation (BSI) should be the highest priority when taking care of patients. Appropriate attire prior to entering the patient's room should include eye protection (goggles), facemask, protective waterproof gown, head cover, and possibly shoe covering should be worn in order to protect against contagious viruses and other organisms in case this patient coughs up blood into the vicinity of health care workers. Assume each and every patient has a dreaded deadly virus (HIV, hepatitis, etc). Treat them according and protect yourself and coworkers.

○ **A dislocation is defined as_____.**

When the articulating surfaces of a joint come out of position, and may result from trauma, diseases that affect the joint, or congenital weaknesses.

○ **Proper nursing evaluation of a dislocated or fracture extremity will include:**

Immobilize and elevate the affected joint/limb, apply ice-water bag as indicated, assess neurovascular status before and after reduction, including strength of pulse, capillary refill time, sensation, movement, pain, and color of skin. With compromised blood areterial flow, a patient may present with the "six Ps": pulses, polar (cold), pain, paresthesia, paralysis, and perfusion.

○ **A radial pulse on exam indicates a BP of at least_____.**

80 mm Hg.

○ **A femoral pulse on exam indicates a BP of at least_____.**

70 mm Hg.

○ **A carotid pulse indicates a BP of at least_____.**

60 mm Hg.

○ **A trauma patient is admitted to the surgical floor. Within the first hour, he is noted to have a decreasing level of consciousness and an enlarging right pupil. What should the nurse suspect?**

Probable uncal herniation with oculomotor nerve compression.

○ **Name five clinical signs of basilar skull fracture.**

Periorbital ecchymosis (raccoon's eyes), retroauricular ecchymosis (Battle sign), otorrhea or rhinorrhea, hemotympanum or bloody ear discharge, and 1st, 2nd, 7th, and 8th CN deficits.

○ **What is the *most common* cause of shock in patients with blunt chest trauma?**

Pelvic or extremity fractures.

○ **What should be checked prior to inserting a chest tube in an intubated patient with respiratory distress and decreased breath sounds on one side?**

Position of the ET tube. One simple formula for calculating the depth or markings at the teeth is to multiply the tube size ×3, which gives the centimeters at the teeth the ET tube should be positioned at. Example: a 7-F endotracheal tube should be inserted, so the markings at the teeth are $7 \times 3 = 21$ cm

○ **A trauma patient is admitted to the medsurg floor. Within the first few hours, a crepitance is detected under the anterior chest skin consistent with subcutaneous emphysema. What should the nurse suspect?**

Pneumothorax or pneumomediastinum; if emphysema is severe, consider a major bronchial injury.

○ **What rib fracture has the worst prognosis?**

First rib. First and second rib fractures are associated with bronchial tears, vascular injury, and myocardial contusions.

○ **What cardiovascular injury is commonly associated with sternal fractures?**

Myocardial contusions (blunt myocardial injury).

○ **Which valve is most commonly injured with blunt trauma?**

Aortic valve.

○ **What is the basic disorder contributing to the pathophysiology of compartment syndrome?**

Damage occurs to muscles or arteries within the muscle compartment. Increased pressure within these closed tissue spaces compromises blood flow to the muscle and nerve tissue. Pressure can be measured using a Stryker or other pressure manometer (art-line setup, etc). Treatment is typically open fasciotomy. There are three prerequisites to the development of compartment syndrome:

(1) Limiting space.

(2) Increased tissue pressure.

(3) Decreased tissue perfusion.

○ **Is the heat of firing significant enough to sterilize a bullet and its wound?**

No, contaminants from clothing, skin body surface, and from viscera can be carried along the bullet's path.

○ **Where are epidural hematomas located?**

Between the dura and inner table of the skull. The most common location is at the thinnest part of the skull near the temporal area, where the middle meningeal artery is most often torn or ruptured resulting in a collection of arterial blood. If large enough, the swelling can cause brain shift and possible death.

○   **Where are subdural hematomas located?**

Beneath the dura and over the brain and arachnoid. Caused by tears of pial arteries or of *bridging veins.* Subdurals typically become symptomatic within 24 hours–2 weeks after injury.

○   **For a trauma victim, which test is most helpful for evaluating retroperitoneal organs?**

CT scan.

○   **What is the most frequently injured organ with blunt trauma?**

Spleen.

○   **What is Kehr's sign?**

Left shoulder pain with splenic rupture. This is due to the innervation of the diaphragm which may be irritated by the blood, causing referred pain to the C-3, 4, 5 dermatomes of the shoulder.

○   **What type of injury most commonly damages the pancreas?**

Penetrating trauma.

○   **Inability to pass a nasogastric tube in a trauma victim suggests damage to what organ?**

Diaphragm, usually on the left.

○   **What type of contrast medium should be used to evaluate the esophagus if traumatic injury is suspected?**

Gastrograffin. If barium is used, it may leak out into the mediastinum or abdomen causing a severe reaction, pain, and scarring.

○   **A stress fracture is suspected of the 2nd or 3rd metatarsal, but none is found on initial x-rays. How long before a 2nd set of x-rays will likely be positive?**

14–21 days.

○   **What is the dose of methylprednisolone used to treat acute spinal cord injury?**

30 mg/kg load over 15 minutes in the 1st h followed by 5.4 mg/kg per hour over the next 23 hours.

  Nurses should check with the neurosurgeon to determine if/when the steroid should be given. There is some controversy about the use of methylprednisolone that may limit its use.

○   **Describe the key features of spinal shock.**

Sudden areflexia which is transient and distal which lasts hours to weeks. BP is usually 80–100 mm Hg with paradoxical bradycardia.

○   **What are the two most commonly injured genitourinary organs?**

(**1**) Kidney.

(**2**) Bladder (associated with pelvic fracture).

○   **A pneumatic tourniquet can be inflated on an extremity to more than a patient's systolic blood pressure for how long?**

2 hours without damage to underlying vessels or nerves.

○ **For how long can wound care be delayed before proliferation of bacteria that may result in infection?**

3 hours.

○ **What mechanisms of injury create wounds that are most susceptible to infection?**

Compression or tension injuries. They are 100 times more susceptible to infection.

○ **What methods has been proven to decrease the pain of local anesthetic administration?**

Buffering the lidocaine solution with sodium bicarbonate, decreasing the speed of injection and use of a subdermal injection instead of superficial or intradermal injections. Bupivicaine and mepivicaine should not be buffered as the bicarbonate may precipitate the anesthesia chemical.

○ **Why is epinephrine added to local anesthesia?**

To increase the duration of the anesthesia (vasoconstriction decreases the rate of absorption). Epinephrine also causes vasoconstriction and decreased bleeding. It may weaken tissue defenses and increases the incidence of wound infection.

○ **How should hair be removed prior to wound repair?**

By clipping the hair around the wound, not by using razor preparation which increases infection rates.

○ **What factors increase the likelihood of wound infection?**

Dirty or contaminated wounds, stellate or crushing wounds, wounds longer than 5 cm, wounds older than 6 hours, retained foreign bodies, and infection prone anatomic sites.

○ **Which has greater resistance to infection, sutures or staples?**

Staples.

○ **What types of wounds result in majority of tetanus cases?**

Lacerations, punctures, crush injuries.

○ **Characterize tetanus prone wounds.**

Age of wound: >6 hours
Configuration: stellate wound.
Depth: >1 cm.
Mechanism of injury: missile, crush, burn, frostbite.
Signs of infection: present.
Devitalized tissue: present.
Contaminants: present.
Denervated and/or ischemic tissue: present.

○ **T/F: It is acceptable to clip or shave an eyebrow if needed to repair the skin.**

False. Eyebrows are valuable landmarks. 15% will not ever regrow.

○ **If a patient has been burned over his entire back, both legs, and right arm, what percentage of his body is considered to be burned?**

63%. Burn percentages are calculated through the rule of 9s:

Face : 9%

Arms : 9% each

Front : 18%

Back : 18%

Legs : 18% each

○ **What life threatening injury is associated with pelvic fractures?**

Severe hemorrhage, usually retroperitoneal or intraperitoneal. Up to 6 liters of blood can be accommodated in this space. Treatment may include stabilization of the fracture (internal or external fixators) and interventional radiology placement of material inside arteries to stop bleeding (embolize).

○ **Define the properties and values in the Glasgow Coma Scale.**

Eye Opening	Verbal Activity	Motor Activity
4. Spontaneous	5. Oriented	6. Obeys command
3. To command	4. Confused	5. Localizes pain
2. To pain	3. Inappropriate	4. Withdraws to pain
1. None	2. Incomprehensible	3. Flexion to pain
	1. None	2. Extension to pain
		1. None

A normal person has a GCS of 15. A dead person has a GCS of 3.

○ **What is the currently approved emergency replacement therapy for massive hemorrhage?**

Type-specific, uncross-matched blood (available in 10–15 minutes). Type O negative, whereas immediately life-saving in certain situations, carries the risk of life-threatening transfusion reactions.

○ **What is the *most common* mechanism of injury in the elderly?**

Falls > MVA > Burns > Assaults.

○ **What formula should be used to calculate the fluid requirements for resuscitation of a burn victim?**

4 ml/kg/% of total body surface area/day. One-half of this is given in the first 8 hours, the other one-half over the next 16 hours (known as the Parkland formula).

○ **Trauma victims are often denied narcotics until what condition is ruled out?**

A closed head injury.

○ **Why is mannitol sometimes given in the treatment of head injuries?**

It is a powerful diuretic that will help reduce cerebral edema.

○ **A trauma victim is admitted to medsurg following an MVA. A physician diagnosed a C-4 fracture and suddenly the patient's BP drops and his pulse slows. What could be a possible cause for these symptoms?**

Spinal shock related to spinal cord injury.

○ **A client is admitted to the floor with a C-6 neck fracture. In what position should the patient be maintained?**

Supine with the head and neck midline and immobilized.

○ **What type of breath sounds will you hear when a pneumothorax is present?**

Decreased or absent breath sounds on the affected side with a collapsed lung.

○ **To prevent increased intercranial pressure in a patient with a head injury, what position should the head of the bed be in?**

Avoid neck flexion, and position the patient with the head of the bed elevated 30 degrees.

○ **After giving the drug mannitol (Osmitrol) to a patient with a head injury, what would be his/her expected urine output?**

It should increase dramatically.

○ **In a trauma victim, what initial assessment should receive the highest priority?**

Establishing an open airway.

○ **A patient was admitted to the hospital with multiple gunshot wounds. The physician determines that this patient requires emergency surgery, or he will die. However, the patient is unconscious and, therefore, is unable to sign the consent forms. No relatives can be found to give consent either. Can this surgery be performed?**

Yes. If the physician determines that the surgery is necessary to save the patient's life, it can be performed without consent.

○ **During a trauma exam, you note that a patient has one pupil that is larger than the other. Pressure on what cranial nerve is involved in producing this symptom?**

The third cranial nerve.

○ **What is the primary cause of new onset seizures in adults over the age of 20?**

Trauma.

○ **A patient has fallen out of their medsurg bed after becoming confused and climbing up and over the rails. What would be a priority concern before moving this patient?**

Possible head trauma and/or spine injury with spinal cord injury requiring head and neck immobilization.

○ **How long can spinal shock last following a spinal cord injury?**

It can last for several weeks after the initial injury.

○   **What is the procedure for the emergency treatment of a burn victim?**

Assess the ABCs, apply sterile sheets to the burned area, and remove smoldering clothing. Use IV fluids to rehydrate the patient using the Parkland formula (above).

○   **What are the signs and symptoms of a pneumothorax?**

Tachypnea, restlessness, hypotension, dyspnea, absent or diminished breath sounds, and possible hypoxia.

○   **What are the signs and symptoms of hypovolemia?**

Rapid weak pulse, low blood pressure, cool clammy skin, shallow respirations, oliguria or anuria, and lethargy.

○   **What is "Battle sign?**

Bluish discolorations (bruising, or subQ blood extravasated) behind the ears of patients who have sustained a basilar skull fracture.

○   **What parts of the skin are affected in a partial thickness burn?**

The epidermis and superficial aspect of the dermis.

○   **How should neurogenic shock be best managed?**

Neurogenic shock is treated with replacement of volume deficit followed by vasopressors (such as neosynephrine).

○   **A patient has an orbital floor fracture; what symptoms and signs might be seen?**

The most common symptom would be diplopia due to entrapment of the inferior rectus and inferior oblique muscles and resultant paralysis of upward gaze. In addition, one would worry that the inferior orbital nerve could be damaged with paresthesia resulting to the lower lid, infraorbital area, and side of the nose.

○   **Is the stomach more commonly injured with penetrating trauma or blunt trauma?**

The stomach is more commonly injured with penetrating trauma.

○   **What is the *most common* body area affected in trauma that results in death?**
The head.

○   **What is the *most common* cause of airway obstruction in trauma?**

CNS depression.

○   **What is the *most common* wound associated with pericardial tamponade?**

Right ventricular injury. It is closest to the anterior chest wall and is most commonly injured by frontal knife and bullet wounds.

○   **What are the signs and symptoms of acute pericardial tamponade?**

Triad of hypotension, elevated CVP, and tachycardia is usually indicative of either acute pericardial tamponade or a tension pneumothorax in a traumatized patient. Muffled heart tones may be auscultated.

○   **What EKG finding is pathognomonic of pericardial tamponade?**

Total electrical alternans. Pulsus paradoxus is nonspecific. Muffled heart tones are subjective findings and are difficult to appreciate.

○   **Name two retroperitoneal organs which may be injured without producing a positive DPL (diagnostic peritoneal lavage).**

Pancreas and duodenum. These are retroperitoneal in location and therefore the blood and amylase/lipase will be difficult to detect as the DPL does not involve the retroperitoneum.

○   **Name two organs that tend to not bleed enough to produce a positive DPL when injured.**

Bladder and small bowel.

○   **What RBC count is considered positive in peritoneal lavage fluid analysis of a patient with blunt abdominal trauma?**

RBC counts of more than 100,000 per mm^3 are considered positive for both penetrating and blunt trauma to the abdomen. 5,000 RBCs per mm^3 is considered positive in a patient with low chest or high abdominal penetrating trauma where diaphragmatic perforation is a possibility.

○   **What is the cause of death secondary to an untreated tension pneumothorax?**

Decreased cardiac output. The vena cava is compressed resulting in decreased right heart blood return and concomitant severe compromise in stroke volume, blood pressure, and cardiac output. Cardiac arrhythmias can also occur. V-tach in a young apparently healthy person is due to a tension pneumothorax until proven otherwise.

○   **Signs of tension pneumothorax on physical exam include:**

Tachypnea, unilateral absent breath sounds, tachycardia, pallor, diaphoresis, cyanosis, tracheal deviation, hypotension, and neck vein distension.

○   **What is the best method to open an airway while maintaining C-spine precautions?**

Jaw thrust.

○   **Describe a patient with a central cord syndrome.**

Injury to the ligamentum flavum and to the cord causing upper extremity neurologic deficit greater than lower extremity deficit. In some patients, the arms will be weak, while the legs may be normal.

○   **Describe a patient with anterior cord syndrome.**

Complete motor paralysis and loss of pain and temperature sensation distal to the lesion.
Posterior column sparing results in intact proprioception and vibration sense.
Causes occlusion of the anterior spinal artery or protrusion of fracture fragments into the anterior canal.

○   **How may a posterior urethral tear be diagnosed in a male?**

High riding, boggy prostate on rectal exam suggests this injury. Blood at the meatus may be present. A Foley catheter should never be placed in a patient with blood at the meatus until it has been okayed by radiology testing (retrograde urethrogram or other test).

○ **What is the mechanism of a posterior urethral tear?**

Associated with pelvic fracture, urethral stricture, impotence, and incontinence.

○ **A patient has a pelvic fracture with suspected bladder or ureteral injury. What test should be performed first, a cystogram or an intravenous pyelogram (IVP)?**

When a pelvic fracture is present or suspected, the cystogram is usually performed first so that distal ureteral dye from the IVP will not mimic extravasation from the bladder.

○ **What is the mechanism of injury responsible for the greatest portion of injuries in the elderly?**

Falls. Most falls are caused by tripping, but other medical causes underlying the initial fall should always be sought.

○ **The organ most severely affected in a blast injury:**

The lungs.

○ **The organ most commonly affected in a blast injury:**

The ears. If the blast victims have blood coming from their ears (ruptured tympanic membranes), they have a 50% chance of a serious internal blast injury.

○ **A trauma patient is admitted to the medsurg floor. She has a closed head injury with suspected elevated intracranial pressure. What treatments should be considered?**

(1) Paralyze the patient and ventilate normally. Do not hyperventilate unless the victim is decompensating/bradycardic and hypotensive with impending brain herniation; excessive hyperventilation will lower PC02 and vasocontrict the brain arteries, causing worsening symptoms and brain injury.

(2) Maintain normal fluid volume (avoid excess fluids).

(3) Elevate the head of the bed to 30 degrees after the C-spine has been cleared.

(4) Consider mannitol 500 ml of a 20% solution over 20 minutes for a 70 kg adult.

Use of diuretics like furosemide is controversial. Steroids are no longer recommended. Barbiturate use is also not recommended. Mannitol use is also losing favor except in cases with sudden deterioration and suspected impending brain herniation.

○ **What should be done prior to insertion of a Foley catheter in a patient with a known pelvic fracture?**

Assess for possible urethral tear injuries—perineal bruising and blood at the meatus are potential signs. Radiological tests may be indicated to prove that there is not a urethral or GU injury. Also, a rectal exam should be done.

○ **When monitoring a pregnant female trauma victim, which vital signs are more likely to indicate hemodynamic instability—the mother's or those of the fetus?**

The fetal heart rate is more sensitive to inadequate resuscitation. Remember that the mother may lose 10–20% of her blood volume without change in vital signs whereas the baby's heart rate may increase or decrease above 160 or below 120 indicating significant fetal distress.

○ **An unconscious, 60-year-old patient is stabilized and admitted to the medsurg floor with a head injury. An ECG shows significant ST segment elevation. What is your concern?**

Although MI should be considered, don't forget the possibility of an intracerebral hemorrhage. This may also cause significant ST segment elevation.

○   **What are the National Institutes of Health treatment recommendations for spinal cord injury?**

Consider giving high dose methylprednisolone (Solu-Medrol) 30 mg/kg bolus over 15 minutes followed by 45 minutes normal saline drip. Over the subsequent 23 hours, the patient should receive an infusion of 5.4 mg/kg/hour of methylprednisolone. Note that this is highly controversial and some neurosurgeons may choose not to give steroids.

○   **A trauma patient presents with a complaint of severe burning pain in the upper extremities and associated neck pain. On physical exam, the patient has good strength in his upper extremities and no obvious neurologic deficits in the lower extremities. Although the C-spine series is negative, what problem is still suspected?**

Central cord syndrome. This injury is due to hyperextension of the spinal cord.

Diagnostic findings include upper extremity neurologic symptoms and minimal or no lower extremity symptoms. Tingling, paresthesias, burning pain, and severe weakness or paralysis in the upper extremities with little or no symptoms in the lower extremities.

○   **A patient is admitted for observation overnight after an MVA (motor vehicle accident) with a history of high speed traumatic injury to the chest. His initial exam per report was normal. On the medsurg floor, your physical exam reveals a systolic murmur over the precordium auscultated. The patient has a slightly hoarse voice, and worsening chest pain. The pulse is also stronger in the upper extremities. What do you suspect?**

Traumatic rupture of the aorta.

○   **What are the two basic mechanisms for elevated compartment pressure?**

(1) External compression—by burn eschar, circumferential casts, dressings, or pneumatic pressure garments.

(2) Volume increase within the compartment—hemorrhage into the compartment, IV infiltration, or edema due to postischemic swelling.

○   **Which two fractures are most commonly associated with compartment syndrome?**

Tibia (resulting most often in anterior compartment involvement) and supracondylar humerus fractures.

○   **What are the early general signs and symptoms of compartment syndrome?**

Early findings: (1) Tenderness and pain out of proportion to the injury, (2) pain with active and passive motion, and (3) hypesthesia (paresthesia)—abnormal 2-point discrimination. Late findings: (1) Compartment tense, indurated, and erythematous, (2) slow capillary refill, and (3) pallor and pulselessness.

○   **A patient is admitted with a tibia fracture and a cast is placed by the orthopedic surgeon. The patient complaints of pain, and the medsurg nurse elevates the leg appropriately, but soon the pain is even worse. What should be suspected?**

Compartment syndrome. Pain is the most common symptom of compartment syndrome due to tissue ischemia. Elevating the limb decreases arterial circulation, thus the pain is worsened in these patients (normally it will decrease pain in patients with uncomplicated fractures). The doctor should be notified immediately and a thorough neurovascular exam will likely be abnormal. Removal of the cast is indicated along with possible surgery to decompress the lower leg compartments.

○   **Following a fall, a patient is admitted and observed, with a swollen, bruised wrist. A possible fracture is suspected. What should you assess in relation to this?**

Assess the area distal to the possible fracture for signs of neurovascular compromise.

○ **What is a stress fracture?**

A stress or "fatigue" fracture is caused by small, repetitive forces, usually involving the metatarsal shafts, the distal tibia, or the femoral neck. These fractures may not be seen on initial radiographs.

○ **A client has a C-6 neck fracture. In what position should the patient be maintained?**

Supine with the head and neck midline and immobilized.

○ **Following casting, what would be the first symptom that would alert you to possible compartment syndrome?**

Pain that is disproportionate to the injury.

○ **What physical findings are typical for a patient with a hip fracture?**

The leg on the affected side is usually shorter, it is abducted and externally rotated, and pain is present.

○ **A trauma patient who is semicomatose is brought to the surgical floor and the nurse notices crepitus, or a gritting sensation whenever they palpate and move the right upper arm. What does this mean?**

Crepitation is used to describe the feeling of bone fragments rubbing together when a fracture is present. An x-ray will likely reveal a fracture.

○ **What are the "five Ps" of compartment syndrome?**

Pain, pallor, pulselessness, paresthesias, and paralysis.

○ **What is the difference between a closed versus an open fracture?**

A closed fracture has the nearby skin intact. An open fracture is a broken bone with the nearby skin lacerated, punctured, or otherwise injured so that bacteria can potentially contaminate the bone fracture site. A sharp bone fragment may lacerate or puncture the skin. Open fractures represent a surgical emergency and ideally these patients are taken to the OR for thorough debridement and cleansing to decrease the chance of osteomyelitis and other infections.

○ **What is a greenstick fracture?**

A fracture in which a break in only one cortex of the bone occurs, usually due to minor or indirect force. The x-ray shows the fracture through about one-half of the bone, with the cortex intact on the other side.

○ **What is a transverse fracture? What is an oblique fracture? What is a spiral fracture?**

A transverse fracture that is at approximately a 90 degree angle to the bone, extending horizontally through the bone. An oblique fracture extends at an oblique angle across both cortices of the bone. A spiral fracture is a fracture that curves around both cortices, and is usually due to twisting force, with the distal part of the bone held or unable to move.

○ **What is the purpose of traction in regards to a fracture?**

To realign bone fragments, decrease pain, decrease neurovascular injury, and to decrease the potential space around the fracture by pulling the proximal and distal bone fragments apart which increases the muscle tension and resulting in less bleeding. A closed femur fracture can cause up to 1 l of blood loss internally if not stabilized and traction applied.

○   **What is your role in regard to maintaining traction in a patient?**

Make sure the weights hang freely, are properly positioned, and the patient is in the proper position in bed.

○   **What is the *most common* fracture in the elderly?**

Hip fracture.

○   **What is the *most common* long bone fracture?**

The tibia.

○   **Most common shoulder dislocation?**

Anterior (95%).

○   **A patient cannot actively abduct her shoulder. What injury does this suggest?**

Rotator cuff tear. The cuff comprises the supraspinatus, infraspinatus, subscapularis, and the teres minor muscles and tendons.

○   **How long after a fracture does a callus start to form?**

5–7 days.

○   **What is the *most common* Salter-Harris class fracture?**

Type II. A triangular fracture involving the metaphysis and an epiphyseal separation.

○   **What is the *most common* metatarsal fracture?**

5th.

○   **What is the *most common* mechanism for fractures of the femoral condyles?**

Direct trauma, fall or blow to the distal femur.

○   **Why would a physician perform an arthrocentesis on a knee with a severe acute hemarthrosis?**

Relieve pressure and pain and to help diagnosis if fat globules are present indicating a fracture.

○   **Who gets Achilles' tendon rupture?**

Middle aged men who play weekend sports occasionally; occurs most commonly on the left side.

○   **What is the *most common* ankle injury?**

75% of ankle injuries are sprains, with 90% of these involving the lateral complex.

90% of lateral ligament injuries are *anterior talofibular*.

○   **How are sprains classified?**

1st—*stretching* of ligament, normal x-ray.

2nd—severe stretching with *partial tear*, marked tenderness, swelling, pain, normal x-ray (now stressed).

3rd—complete ligament *rupture*, marked tenderness, swelling, and obviously deformed joint. X-ray may show an abnormal joint.

○ **What is unique about avulsion fractures at the base of the fifth metatarsal?**

It is one of the most commonly missed fractures, history is of ankle injury from plantar flexion and inversion.

○ **Describe the leg position in a patient with an anterior hip dislocation.**

Hip is abducted and externally rotated. 10% of hip dislocations. Mechanism is forced abduction. If anterior superior, hip is extended. If anterior inferior, hip is flexed.

○ **Describe the leg position in a patient with a posterior hip dislocation.**

Shortened, adducted, and internally rotated. 90% of hip dislocations. Force applied to a flexed knee directed posteriorly (commonly from a car accident with dashboard injury). Associated with sciatic nerve injury (10%) and avascular necrosis of the femoral head.

○ **What is the appropriate initial nursing intervention when caring for an open wound near a fracture?**

Grossly decontaminate, rinse briefly with sterile saline, then cover with wet sterile dressings.

○ **After application of a traction splint to a femur fracture, what should the nurse assess?**

Check the neurovascular status distal to the fracture. Monitor for skin condition and avoid complications of excessive pressure.

○ **Describe the appropriate basic care of an amputated body part.**

Gently clean to remove debris, wrap in normal saline soaked gauze, place in plastic bag, and seal and place on a solution of ice and water. Do not allow the part to freeze, or to become macerated. Do not place directly on ice as the temperature is usually 10 degrees below freezing and may cause frostbite or tissue damage. The part must also be labeled and placed/transported with the patient.

○ **What is therational for the initial immobilization of a fracture?**

To prevent damage to blood vessels, tissues and nerves, and also to decrease pain level.

○ **What are the four basic treatment components when treating muscle strains and ligament sprains?**

Rest, ice, compression dressing, and elevation. The mnemonic is "RICE." The temperature of ice is often below freezing and could cause frostbite. Therefore, ice should be placed in a bag with water, and applied in contact with the injured area, alternating 20 minutes on and 20 minutes off for most of the first 24 hours. Following this, moist heat and gently increasing range of motion exercises and stretching will aid in healing and recovery. Prolonged immobilization is unnecessary and potentially harmful.

○ **What is the term that describes the inflammation of the synovial cavity surrounding a joint?**

Bursitis.

○ **A medsurg nurse is taking care of a patient with multiple fractures including a femur fracture. The patient develops confusion, shortness of breath, faster breathing and tachycardia, hypotension, and petechiae about 12 hours after admission. What syndrome is likely developing?**

Fat embolism syndrome, where the fat from inside of the bone migrates to the vein, back to the heart and embolizes throughout the body. Symptoms may be minor or may result in ARDS and death.

○ **How soon can fat embolism syndrome occur following a long bone fracture?**

12–72 hours.

○ **What would be a priority nursing intervention for a client with fat embolism syndrome?**

Ensure adequate oxygenation and ventilation due to the impaired gas exchange . . . shortness of breath, abnormal x-ray of lung may be found. Contact the physician, consider transfer to the ICU.

○ **What are key nursing considerations for patients in skeletal or skin traction when being treated for fractures?**

Check the entire traction setup, pin sites, and all suspension apparatus for signs of loosening or excessive tension. Ensure that weight/traction is constant, including during nursing care, check all skin surfaces for signs of pressure, and provide physical and psychological comfort.

○ **A medsurg nurse is examing a nursing home patient who is admitted with confusion and dehydration. The nurse notes that the patient's right leg is shorter than the other leg, is externally rotated, and the patient moans when the lower leg is moved. The likely diagnosis is _____.**

Hip fracture

○ **What is the age group that has the highest hip fracture rate?**

Elderly, especially older women who are at risk for falls and have osteoporosis.

○ **What is the difference between intracapsular hip fracture vs extracapsular?**

Intracapsular hip fractures are those of the femoral head and neck, which are inside the hip capsule (ligaments around joint). Extracapsular fractures involve the femoral trochanteric and shaft and are outside of the capsule.

○ **A medsurg nurse preparing a patient for surgery of the hip fracture. What important steps should be performed?**

Monitor vital signs, watching for hypotension as up to 1,000 cc of blood can be lost into the femur or hip fracture. Monitor for hypothermia and other complications of trauma. Ensure the pre-op medical screening is completed by the physician, along with appropriate tests. Keep pt NPO, have the patient empty the bladder or place Foley catheter. Send an abduction pillow to the OR if indicated, as it is used to keep prosthetic hip joints in proper position. Ensure proper tetanus immunization. Ensure that the consent form is signed after the doctor discusses the plan and operation with patient and family. Arrange for preoperative antibiotics if ordered. If a transfusion of blood is needed, then take a time-out and ensure that the patient is properly matched.

○ **A medsurg nurse taking care of a post-op hip fracture patient should ensure what important steps?**

Monitor vital signs and neurovascular status, watch for signs of post-op bleeding and infection, perform dressing changes, watch for possible fat or pulmonary embolism, administer appropriate anticoagulant and use external pneumatic compression devices/stockings; monitor wound drainage, position limb appropriately (abduction if a prosthesis was used, neutral if not), turn patient, encourage deep breathing and coughing often, use incentive spirometer every hour while awake, monitor I and Os, get the patient to exercise in bed and get up and active as soon as the surgeon allows, control pain, teach the patient proper use of walker/appropriate weight-bearing, and provide support for the patient and family members. Arrange appropriate discharge and ensure adequate supplies and support for the patient when they return home.

○ **A patient in balances suspension traction for a fractured femur needs repositioning toward the head of the bed. What is the proper technique regarding the traction when moving the patient?**

Maintain the same degrees of traction tension . . . do not release or lift the traction during repositioning.

○ **T/F: When teaching the patient crutch walking, all the weight should be placed in the hands rather than the axilla.**

True. Placing pressure on the axilla could cause nerves damage.

○ **Lower back pain is usually caused by _____. Describe risk factors for this.**

Musculoskeletal strains/sprain. Risk factors include obesity, poor body mechanisms, and lifting of heavy objects.

○ **A medsurg nurse should consider what serious problems in any patient who suddenly complaints of back pain?**

Abdominal aortic aneurysm, cauda equina syndrome (compression of lower spinal nerves), tumor or acute bleed into the spinal column or peritoneum, bowel infarction, kidney stone or infection, and others.

○ **What is osteoarthritis?**

A noninflammatory joint disease causing degenerative changes in the articular cartilage, affecting weight-bearing joints including the hips, knees, and vertebrae, as well as possibly any other joint.

○ **How does obesity affect the development of osteoarthritis?**

Osteoarthritis is a degenerative joint disease caused by the wear and tear on weight bearing joints. Obesity increases this wear and tear, and can worsen osteoarthritis.

○ **What is osteomyelitis?**

An acute or chronic infection of the bone or bone marrow, usually affecting the long bones (femur, tibia, humerus), and vertebrae, but an infection can arise in any bone, especially with recent local trauma. Long-term antibiotics (6 weeks or more) and possible surgery are required for treatment.

○ **What is the *most common* cause of infection in bones (osteomyelitis)?**

Staphylococcus aureus (90%)

○ **What is osteoporosis?**

A systemic disease in which bone mass and bone density decrease because of a disturbance in the balance between bone resorption and bone deposition. It may begin as early as age 30, but progresses rapidly after age 45–50. Seventy percent of women older than age 45 have osteoporosis. These people are at increased risk of bone fracture and chronic pain. A common cause is inadequate dietary intake of calcium. After age 35, women cannot add calcium to their bones . . . inadequate ingestion of calcium results in the body taking calcium from the bones which can never be replaced.

○ **What are the causes of osteoporosis?**

Insufficient intake of calcium and vitamin D, smoking, menopausal decreases in estrogen, immobility, long-term steroid use, and caffeine/soda intake.

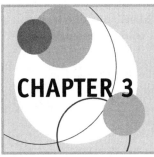

CHAPTER 3

Eyes, Ears, Nose, and Throat (EENT) Pearls

○ **A 34-year-old female patient is admitted to the medical floor with an altered level of consciousness. On day 2, she awakens and complaints of pain in the jaw, she also has a burning sensation in the roof of her mouth, pain when opening the mouth, and an earache. On exam, crepitus is present as well as tenderness over the mandible joint capsule. Diagnosis?**

TMJ syndrome.

○ **What is the resultant deformity if an auricular (ear) hematoma is not properly treated?**

Cauliflower ear.

○ **A patient is seen with herpetic lesions on the tip of the nose. Why is this a problem?**

The tip of the nose and the cornea are both supplied by the nasociliary nerve. Thus, the cornea may also be involved. Untreated herpes infection of the cornea can lead to visual problems and severe complications. Urgent ophthalmology consultation is indicated.

○ **A patient presents with an itching, tearing, right eye. On exam, huge cobblestone papillae are found under the upper lid. Diagnosis?**

Allergic conjunctivitis.

○ **A patient presents with inflammation of the conjunctiva and lid margins. Slit-lamp exam reveals a "greasy" appearance of lid margins with scaling, especially around the base of the lashes. Diagnosis?**

Blepharitis. Often caused by staphylococcal infection of the oil glands and skin next to the lash follicles. Treatment consists of scrubbing with baby shampoo and, in consultation with an ophthalmologist, sulfacetamide drops and a steroid.

○ **A patient admitted for abdominal pain also complains of a pustular vesicle at the lid margin. What would you suspect and how is it treated?**

Hordeolum (stye). Acute inflammation of the meibomian gland, most commonly of the upper lid. Treat with topical antibiotics and warm compresses. Surgical drainage may be necessary.

○ **A patient presents with a chronic nontender uninflamed nodule of the upper lid. What would you suspect?**

Chalazion. Usually treated by surgical curettage.

○ **A patient admitted with a headache on day 3 complains of a sudden abnormal vision and partial loss of vision in one eye. Physical exam demonstrates a loss of central vision, peripheral vision is preserved. Diagnosis?**

Retrobulbar neuritis. 25% of cases of retrobulbar neuritis are associated with MS (multiple sclerosis).

○ **A patient presents with sudden loss of vision in one eye which returned quickly. Diagnosis?**

Amaurosis fugax. Usually caused by central retinal artery emboli from extracranial atherosclerosis. A thorough neurological evaluation/consultation is indicated, including likely an MRI of the brain and evaluating of carotid arteries. The next time an emboli occurs, it may result in a major stroke.

○ **A patient presents with the sensation of painless loss of vision in one eye described as a wall slowly developing in the visual field. Findings expected on ophthalmoscopic exam?**

Gray detached retina. Patient may also complain of flashing lights in the peripheral visual field or "spider webs" in the visual field. Inferior detachment is treated with the patient sitting up. Superior detachment is treated with the patient lying flat.

○ **What are the causes of retinal detachment?**

Primary retinal detachment is due to a change in the retina or vitreous humor; a secondary detachment results from inflammation or trauma. Treatment is usually indicated, including heat (diathermy), laser, cryotherapy, or scleral buckling (band around eyeball).

○ **What are pre- and postoperative nursing interventions for patients with a retinal detachment?**

Bed rest, patch the eye as prescribed (one or both), position the patient's head so that the retinal tear (or hole) is at the lowest point of the eye (downward) to prevent enlargement or further detachment. Cleanse face, give antibiotics and eye drops pre-op, sign permit, support patient and family and ease their fears about potential loss of vision. Postoperative instructions include review of postoperative instructions carefully, as the patient will likely not be able to read due to visual impairment. Patient should not bend, strain, cough, rub eyes, or strain at bowel movements (increases intraocular pressure). No quick movements or strenuous physical activities/sports until healed. Close followup and return for any complications.

○ **A patient is admitted to surgery with a history of being struck in the eye during a violent MVA. The patient is admitted with a femur fracture and also has eye trauma. On exam, no abnormalities are evident. What should the patient be told?**

Inform the nurse if ocular pain or blurred vision develops. Repeat exam within 24 hours. Hyphema caused by blunt eye trauma may not be present on initial exam. Retinal detachments may slowly occur and patients should tell medical staff if abnormal vision develops.

○ **What are miotic eye drops used to treat?**

Glaucoma. Pilocarpine is the most common, instilled 4 times daily.

○ **For treatment of glaucoma, what is the function of acetazolamide and glycerol?**

Acetazolamide—carbonic anhydrase inhibitor; decreases ciliary body aqueous output. Glycerol—hyperosmotic agent; decreases intraocular pressure by making plasma hypertonic to aqueous humor.

○ **A 48-year-old diabetic male with DKA is hospitalized. He says he was wondering about the pain, itching, and discharge from the right ear. On exam, the eardrum is intact. The external ear canal is red and narrow and inflamed. What is your diagnosis?**

Otitis externa. Treat by removing debris from ear canal, treating for one week with an antibiotic-steroid otic solution. For severe narrowing of canal, an earwick may be used for 2–3 days to improve delivery of antibiotic. Diabetics are at higher risk of malignant external otitis, which is a severe ear infection with involvement of bone near the canal.

○ **What potential complication of a nasal fracture should always be considered on physical exam?**

Septal hematoma. If not drained, aseptic necrosis of the septal cartilage or septal abscess may develop.

○ **In what age group are peritonsillar abscesses *most common*?**

Adolescents and young adults. Symptoms may include ear pain, trismus, drooling, and alteration of voice.

○ **A patient presents 3 days after tooth extraction with severe pain and a foul mouth odor and taste. What complication does the patient most likely have?**

Alveolar osteitis (dry socket). Treat by irrigation of the socket, medicated dental packing, or iodoform with Campho-Phenique or eugenol.

○ **Describe the symptoms of acute necrotizing ulcerative gingivitis.**

Gingival pain and foul odor and taste in the mouth. On exam, fever and lymphadenopathy are present. The gingiva is bright red and the papillae are ulcerated and covered with a gray membrane.

○ **A 47-year-old female on the medical floor complains of excruciating sudden waxing and waning pain in the right cheek. She says it feels like an electric shock. What disorder does this describe?**

Tic douloureux.

○ **What are the signs and symptoms of a mandibular fracture?**

Malocclusion, pain, decreased range of motion, bony deformity, swelling, ecchymosis, and mental nerve anesthesia. The teeth may be offset, and lacerations of the gums with bleeding may be seen.

○ **What is the *most common* type of mandibular fracture?**

Alveolar (tooth-bearing segment of the mandible). Numbness of the lower lip suggests a mandibular fracture.

○ **Signs and symptoms of fracture of the zygomaticomaxillary complex?**

Emphysema of the tissue, edema, ecchymosis, facial flattening, unilateral epistaxis, anesthesia, step deformity, decreased mandibular movement, and diplopia.

○ **What are the two *most common* findings with an orbital floor injury?**

Diplopia and globe lowering.

○ **What methods can be used for the emergency storage of an avulsed tooth?**

The tooth can be placed in a small container of milk, or the patient may place the tooth underneath his/her tongue. Several companies make a first-aid solution in a small cup that may be used as well for transporting avulsed teeth. Teeth that are out of place for over 1–2 hours are unlikely to successfully be reimplanted and survive.

○ **When should a patient's eye not be dilated?**

When the patient has narrow angle glaucoma or an iris-supported intraocular lens.

○ **Why shouldn't a patient be given for home use any topical ophthalmologic anesthetics?**

These anesthetics inhibit healing and eliminate sensation, thereby decreasing the eye's natural ability to protect itself. Patients may unintentionally rub their eye severely with significant corneal/eye injury painlessly.

○ **What is a hyphema?**

Blood in the anterior chamber of the eye. Keep the head elevated in these patients. Ophthalmology consultation is indicated. Patients are at risk of losing their eyesight entirely if significant bleeding occurs, which may do so 24–48 hours later.

○ **Define strabismus.**

Strabismus is defined as a lack of parallelism of the visual axis of the eyes. Esotropias are medially deviated, exotropias are laterally deviated.

○ **An elderly patient presents with the complaint of seeing halos around lights. What diagnosis is suspected?**

Glaucoma. Another presenting complaint of glaucoma is blurred vision. Also, consider digitalis toxicity.

○ **What effect would you expect phenylephrine hydrochloride (Neosynephrine) drops to have on the eye?**

Mydriasis (pupil dilation).

○ **You would expect intraocular pressure to be affected in what way by administering Neosynephrine eye drops?**

It would increase.

○ **What test can you perform to determine if the drainage from the nose following a head injury is cerebrospinal fluid?**

Test the fluid for glucose using a test strip. If it registers near the normal blood glucose level, then it is likely cerebrospinal fluid. Nasal secretions are lower in glucose than serum glucose.

○ **A common adverse effect of aminoglycoside therapy is what type of neurological damage?**

Damage to the 8th cranial nerve.

○ **What is the medical abbreviation for the left eye?**

"OS". Increasingly, hospitals are changing chart documentation to simply "left eye" or "right eye," and avoiding "OS" and "OD" (right eye).

○ **What is the medical abbreviation for both eyes?**

Oculus Ulterque (OU)

○ **What is the cause of "floaters" commonly seen by patients with a retinal detachment?**

Red blood cells that have been released into the vitreous humor, which move slowly and appear as floating shadows.

○ **Where is the correct site to instill eye drops?**

The lower conjunctival sac.

○ **What effect does a miotic agent have on the pupil?**

It constricts the pupil.

○ **What effect does a mydriatic agent have on the pupil?**

It dilates the pupil.

○ **What is a tonometer?**

A device that measures intraocular pressure.

○ **Why are a patient's eyes patched when a retinal detachment is present?**

It decreases eye movements that could worsen the detachment.

○ **What symptoms does a patient display if he has a retinal detachment?**

Seeing "flashing lights" or "floaters" and a nonpainful loss of vision frequently described as "a curtain slowly drawn across the eye."

○ **What is the first visual disturbance seen with open angle glaucoma?**

Peripheral vision loss.

○ **What type of glaucoma is considered a medical emergency?**

Acute narrow-angle glaucoma.

○ **What is the outcome of an untreated retinal detachment?**

Blindness.

○ **What are the symptoms of narrow angle glaucoma?**

Severe eye pain, rapid vision loss, and colored halos around lights.

○ **Why should an order for atropine be questioned in a patient with glaucoma?**

Atropine causes pupil dilation, which can increase intraocular pressure.

○ **What is the best method for detecting the development of glaucoma?**

Yearly intraocular pressure readings after the age of 40.

○ **What is the purpose of instilling phenylephrine hydrochloride eye drops?**

It acts as a mydriatic and also constricts small blood vessels in the eye.

○ **What is pilocarpine hydrochloride used for?**

Chronic open-angle glaucoma.

○ **How can you prevent medication from entering the tear duct (and draining away) when administering eye drops?**

After instilling the eye drop, apply light pressure against the nose at the inner angle of the patient's closed eye.

○ **What is the normal intraocular pressure?**

12–20 mm Hg. If elevated above this, then suspect glaucoma. A tonometer can be used by medical staff to measure intraocular pressure (IOP).

○ **Before removing a foreign body from a patient's eye, what should you first check?**

The patient's visual acuity.

○ **What are mydriatic drugs used for?**

To dilate the pupils in preparation for an intraocular exam. They are also used to decrease iris muscle spasm in patients with eye infections and decrease photophobia.

○ **How do you remove wax or a foreign body from the ear?**

Gently flush with warm saline solution. A dilute solution of sodium bicarbonate (4–8% approx) placed into the ear 5 minutes prior will loosen the wax considerably and allow easier removal.

○ **When testing the six cardinal fields of gaze, which cranial nerves are being assessed?**

3, 4, and 6.

○ **What is the primary reason for treating streptococcal pharyngitis with antibiotics?**

To protect the heart valves and prevent rheumatic fever.

○ **What is trismus?**

Painful spasms of the muscles of mastication.

○ **What is the treatment for a corneal injury from a caustic substance?**

Flush both eyes with copious amounts of water for 20–30 minutes.

○ **How do you remove a patient's artificial eye?**

Depress the lower lid. The artificial eye is usually a curvilinear piece of glass or plastic that lays against a round prosthesis posteriorly. If possible, allow the patient to perform this or assist.

○ **How do you clean an artificial eye?**

Soap and water.

○ **What is the major complication of Bell's palsy?**

Corneal inflammation (keratitis).

○ **Prior to administering a treatment to the eye, what should the nurse document?**

Visual acuity.

○ **A client is admitted with acute narrow glaucoma. A diuretic is ordered. Why?**

To lower the intraocular pressure.

○ **A patient in triage complains of a sore throat. What further assessment should be done to determine the patient's need for urgent care?**

Assess for difficulty in breathing, swallowing, stridor, fever, or difficulty in talking.

○ **What is an early symptom of laryngeal cancer?**

Hoarseness.

○ **A patient is admitted for severe epistaxis. Initially it stopped, but then soon the blood was flowing significantly from the left nostril. What should be the initial nursing action to control bleeding?**

Have the client sit upright, lean slightly forward, and apply pressure directly by pinching the nostrils.

○ **What finding would lead the nurse to suspect an ear infection in a 1 year old?**

History of fever and pulling at the ear.

○ **A patient is admitted for stridor. Soon the patient develops increasing fever, sore throat, difficulty in speaking, pale color, and drooling. What should the nurse suspect?**

Epiglottitis.

○ **What would a priority nursing diagnosis be for this patient?**

Airway obstruction and ineffective airway clearance.

○ **Why is topical cocaine often used in the treatment of epistaxis?**

It anesthetizes the area and constricts blood vessels, decreasing bleeding. Pharmacies are increasingly avoiding the use of cocaine due to costs and other issues.

○ **A patient is admitted to the floor with a tracheal fracture. After 3 hours, he develops worsening respiratory distress and several attempts at endotracheal intubation fail. What emergency procedure should the nurse prepare for?**

Cricothyroidotomy.

○ **T/F: A cricothyroidotomy may be performed with a large bore, 12 g–14 g needle.**

True.

○ **What is an appropriate nursing diagnosis for the patient with Menière's disease?**

Sensory or perceptual alteration.

○ **T/F: A nasal fracture is a closed fracture.**

False. All nasal fractures should be treated as open fractures.

○ **What are cataracts?**

Loss of transparency of the lens of the eye or its capsule, causing a decrease or loss of vision.

○ **What are the types of cataracts and their causes?**

Congenital cataracts develop in utero and are associated with maternal rubella infection in the first trimester, or hereditary. Complicated cataracts develop due to other diseases (diabetes, glaucoma, retinal detachments, etc.); senile cataracts occur after age 50 as part of aging; toxic cataracts occur from chemical or drug toxicity; traumatic cataracts are caused by mechanical trauma or radiation. Treatment is usually by replacement with plastic intraocular lens implants.

○ **What are important postoperative interventions and instructions after cataract surgery?**

Review postoperative instructions carefully, as the patient will likely not be able to read due to visual impairment. Patient should not bend, strain, cough, rub eyes, or strain at bowel movements (increases intraocular pressure). No quick movements or strenuous physical activities/sports until healed. Close followup and return for any complications.

○ **What otosclerosis?**

Hardening of the ear bones that prevents normal ossicular (ear bone) movement. Runs in families, occurs between ages 15 and 50, women more than men. Treatment is often surgery, with replacement of the stapes.

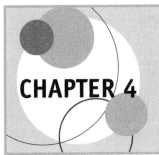

CHAPTER 4 Pulmonary Pearls

○ **What is the *most common* organism causing bacterial pneumonia?**

Pneumococcal pneumoniae.

○ **What percentage of upper respiratory infectious agents are nonbacterial?**

Nonbacterial agents account for over 90% of pharyngitis, laryngitis, tracheal bronchitis, and bronchitis.

○ **Name two antiviral medications that are useful for viral pneumonia.**

Amantadine for influenza A and aerosolized ribavirin for respiratory syncylial virus (RSV).

○ **An older patient with GI symptoms, hyponatremia, and a relative bradycardia most likely has what type of pneumonia?**

Legionella.

○ **What is the medical treatment for Legionella pneumonia?**

IV erythromycin.

○ **Who will benefit from pentamidine prophylactic therapy for PCP (pneumocystis carinii pneumonia)?**

Immunocompromised people with previous history of PCP and those with absolute CD4 (T-helper cells) counts less than 200. Criteria for pentamidine prophylaxis are becoming more relaxed.

○ **What are the classic signs and symptoms of TB?**

Night sweats, fever, weight loss, malaise, cough, and a green/yellow sputum most commonly seen in the mornings.

○ **What are some common extrapulmonary TB sites?**

Lymph node, bone, GI tract, GU tract, meninges, liver, and the pericardium.

○ **Right upper lobe cavitation with parenchymal involvement is classic for:**

TB. Lower lung infiltrates, hilar adenopathy, atelectasis, and pleural effusion are also common.

○ **T/F: People under 35 years of age with positive TB skin tests should have at least 6 months of isoniazid chemoprophylaxis.**

True.

○   **Is there a higher incidence of spontaneous pneumothorax among males or females?**

Males. Especially tall, thin males who smoke.

○   **What accessory x-rays may be obtained to diagnose a pneumothorax?**

(1) Expiratory film and (2) lateral decubitus film with the suspected lung up.

○   **What kind of pneumonias are commonly associated with a pneumothorax?**

Staph, TB, Klebsiella, and PCP.

○   **What laboratory tests aid in the diagnosis of PCP?**

A rising LDH or LDH > 450 and an ESR > 50. A low albumin implies a worse prognosis.

○   **The initial therapy for PCP includes what antibiotics?**

TMP–SMZ or pentamidine.

○   **List two drugs that can cause ARDS.**

Heroin and aspirin.

○   **Are sedatives beneficial in acutely asthmatic patients?**

No. They may be dangerous.

○   **What is a PE?**

Pulmonary embolism, a blockage in the pulmonary artery.

○   **What are the *most common* symptoms and signs of PE?**

Tachypnea (92%)
Chest pain (88%)
Dyspnea (84%)
Anxiety (59%)
Tachycardia (44%)
Fever (43%)
Deep vein thrombosis (32%)
Hypotension (25%)
Syncope (13%)

○   **T/F: Pulse oximetry provides a reliable means of estimating oxyhemoglobin saturation in a patient suffering CO poisoning.**

False. COHb has light absorbance that can lead to a falsely elevated pulse oximeter transduced saturation level. The *calculated* value from a standard ABG may also be falsely elevated. The oxygen saturation should be *measured* using a co-oximeter that *measures* the amounts of unsaturated O_2Hb, of COHb and of MetHb.

○ **What procedures should be performed to prevent aspiration in a patient who is continuously vomiting and at risk for aspiration pneumonia?**

Lie the patient on his right side in the Trendelenburg position. This will help confine the aspiration to the right upper lobe.

○ **Are aspirated foreign bodies more likely to be found in the right or left bronchus?**

The right. This is because the right bronchus is straighter in line with the upper trachea and foreign objects are more likely to follow this path.

○ **Which strain of influenza is more common in adults?**

Adults: Influenza A.

○ **How do steroids function in the treatment of asthma?**

Steroids increase cAMP, decrease inflammation, and aid in restoring the function of responsiveness to adrenergic drugs. Oral, IV, and inhaled steroids all work well in asthma treatment.

○ **A client with right lower lobe pneumonia is admitted, with normal blood pressure and mild tachypnea. Which nursing action takes priority, elevating the head of the bed, or assessing breath sounds?**

Elevating the head of the bed. The patient's comfort and ease in breathing take priority.

○ **A patient with COPD needs oxygen. Which of the following would deliver the most accurate concentration of oxygen: nasal prongs, simple face mask, or Venturi mask?**

A Venturi mask.

○ **A homeless patient is admitted. He complains of night sweats, fever, cough, hemoptysis, pleuritic chest pain, and had a positive PPD skin test. What conclusions can you draw from this data?**

That the patient had been exposed to M. tuberculosis. Further diagnosis of active TB is confirmed by chest x-ray and sputum samples.

○ **Why is it important not to give a COPD client high concentrations of oxygen?**

It will depress the COPD patient's drive to breathe. Patients with long-standing lung disease depend upon the oxygen concentration more than carbon dioxide to drive ventilations. Additional oxygen causes them to slow respirations, build up CO_2, and potentially become less responsive and stop breathing.

○ **What is the mode of transmission for the tubercle bacillus?**

Inhalation of tubercle-laden droplets.

○ **Interpret the following blood gases: pH 7.49, $PaCO_2$ 26, HCO_3 23, PaO_2 100.**

Respiratory alkalosis.

○ **Interpret the following blood gases: pH 7.30, $PaCO_2$ 50, HCO_3 24, PaO_2 80.**

Respiratory acidosis.

○ **You note that there is no bubbling in the suction compartment of the water seal container of a chest tube. What would be your best course of action?**

Check the order to see if the chest tube is ordered with suction and how much. If suction is ordered, increase the suction to the amount ordered.

○ **Why is the administration of propanolol hydrochloride (Inderal) and other beta blockers used cautiously (relative contraindicated) in clients with COPD?**

It can cause increased airway resistance due to beta blockade and increased smooth muscle contraction of the lungs.

○ **What type of lab study is used to determine if the tubercle bacilli is present in sputum?**

Acid-fast staining.

○ **What is the general course of treatment for someone who has a positive Mantoux test, but does not have active TB?**

Oral isoniazid therapy for approximately 9 months.

Patients suspected of having tuberculosis should have appropriate specimens collected for microscopic examination and mycobacterial culture. When the lung is the site of disease, three sputum specimens should be obtained. Sputum induction with hypertonic saline may be necessary to obtain specimens and bronchoscopy (both performed under appropriate infection control measures) may be considered for patients who are unable to produce sputum, depending on the clinical circumstances. Susceptibility testing for INH, RIF, and EMB should be performed on a positive initial culture, regardless of the source of the specimen. Second-line drug susceptibility testing should be done only in reference laboratories and be limited to specimens from patients who have had prior therapy, who are contacts of patients with drug-resistant tuberculosis, who have demonstrated resistance to rifampin or to other first-line drugs, or who have positive cultures after more than 3 months of treatment.

It is recommended that all patients with tuberculosis have counseling and testing for HIV infection, at least by the time treatment is initiated, if not earlier. For patients with HIV infection, a CD4+ lymphocyte count should be obtained. Patients with risk factors for hepatitis B or C viruses (e.g., injection drug use, foreign birth in Asia or Africa, HIV infection) should have serologic tests for these viruses. For all adult patients baseline measurements of serum amino transferases (aspartate aminotransferase [AST], alanine aminotransferase [ALT]), bilirubin, alkaline phosphatase, and serum creatinine and a platelet count should be obtained. Testing of visual acuity and red–green color discrimination should be obtained when EMB is to be used.

○ **What is the treatment usually for someone with active TB?**

Treatment for 6–9 months with isoniazid and rifampin as the first choice; other medicines possibly used include ethambutol, pyrazinamide, and streptomycin. During treatment of patients with pulmonary tuberculosis, a sputum specimen for microscopic examination and culture should be obtained at a minimum of monthly intervals until two consecutive specimens are negative on culture. More frequent AFB smears may be useful to assess the early response to treatment and to provide an indication of infectiousness. For patients with extrapulmonary tuberculosis, the frequency and kinds of evaluations will depend on the site involved. In addition, it is critical that patients have clinical evaluations at least monthly to identify possible adverse effects of the antituberculosis medications and to assess adherence. Generally, patients do not require followup after completion of therapy but should be instructed to seek care promptly if signs or symptoms recur.

Routine measurements of hepatic and renal function and platelet count are not necessary during treatment unless patients have baseline abnormalities or are at increased risk of hepatotoxicity (e.g., hepatitis B or C virus infection, alcohol abuse). At each monthly visit patients taking EMB should be questioned regarding possible visual disturbances including blurred vision or scotomata; monthly testing of visual acuity and color discrimination is recommended for patients taking doses that on a milligram per kilogram basis.

○ **What changes in chest shape would you expect in someone with advanced COPD?**

An increased anterior–posterior diameter or "barrel chest."

○ **What advice should you give to a patient who is on oral birth control and is also taking INH?**

An alternate method of birth control should be used. INH decreases the effectiveness.

○ **What is the overall goal for the nursing diagnosis of impaired gas exchange?**

To promote optimal respiratory ventilation.

○ **What level should the collection and suction bottles from a chest tube be kept at in relation to the patient?**

Below the level of the patient's chest. This prevents fluids from draining down the chest tube back inside the patient which would increase risk of infection, and decrease accuracy of I and Os.

○ **Above what level of oxygen concentration is there an increased risk for causing oxygen toxicity?**

40%.

○ **What is the primary risk factor in the development of COPD?**

Cigarette smoking and second-hand smoke.

○ **A patient with a gunshot wound to the chest is admitted. He has a chest tube inserted and a pleurovac attached. The next day, he becomes increasingly dyspneic, tachycardic, and tachypneic. What should you check for?**

Any signs that may indicate that the chest tube is blocked. Common causes are blood clots, kinks in the tubing, and suction failure.

○ **Why is pursed-lip breathing taught to clients with emphysema?**

It causes a physiologic "PEEP" (positive end-expiratory pressure), which distends the alveoli due to increased alveolar pressure, increasing surface area and this making it easier to gain oxygen and eliminate carbon dioxide.

○ **What is the cause of pleuritic chest pain in pneumonia?**

Friction between the pleural layers caused by movements in the chest during inspiration and expiration. The lung surface is inflamed due to infection, and the pain fibers are sensitized and especially painful with any movement or rubbing.

○ **Why are clients often prescribed at least two drugs for the treatment of tuberculosis?**

It helps in reducing the development of resistant strains of the disease.

○ **What groups of people are at a high risk of developing tuberculosis today?**

The elderly, homeless, immunosuppressed/immunocompromised (AIDS), foreign born from underdeveloped countries, IV drug abusers, and other substance abusers.

○ **A patient is hyperventilating and blood gases are drawn. What results would you expect to see?**

Normal PO_2, decreased PCO_2, increased pH: Respiratory alkalosis.

○   **What is the most accurate method of evaluating whether oxygen therapy is effective for a patient?**

Arterial blood gases.

○   **What is the recommended technique for testing a patient's gag reflex?**

Touch the back of the patient's tongue or throat with a tongue depressor or swab. This should be done cautiously, with suction immediately available in case it causes sudden vomiting.

○   **An unconscious patient becomes restless. What could this indicate?**

Hypoxia. Full evaluation and assessment of the ABCs may reveal the cause.

○   **Why would you hyper oxygenate a patient prior to suctioning his airway?**

To prevent hypoxia resulting from the suctioning procedure.

○   **When suctioning a patient via the trachea or an endotracheal tube, when is suction never applied?**

When inserting the catheter into the airway.

○   **What solution may be instilled into a tracheostomy or endotracheal tube to help liquefy secretions prior to suctioning?**

1–2 ml of sterile normal saline.

○   **Airway suctioning is considered a clean or sterile procedure?**

Sterile.

○   **What constitutes a positive tuberculin test?**

10 mm or more of induration at the injection site.

○   **In a patient with finger clubbing, what pulmonary condition must be suspected?**

COPD.

○   **When should a tuberculin skin test be read?**

48–72 hours after administration if it's a one-step test. Hospitals are now requiring a two-step test for individuals newly hired into a healthcare facility to elicit responses that may be missed with a one-step.

○   **If cyanosis occurs circumorally, sublingually, or in the nail beds, the oxygen saturation is below what level?**

80%.

○   **What are the early signs and symptoms of tuberculosis?**

Low-grade fever, weight loss, night sweats, fatigue, cough, and anorexia.

○   **What is the approximate oxygen concentration of a patient receiving 3 liters of O_2 per nasal cannula?**

32%. Note that room air oxygen concentration is 21%.

○   **What is Cheyne-Stokes respiration?**

Alternating periods of apnea and deep, rapid breathing. There are multiple causes. A serious intracranial abnormality such as acute bleeding or tumor should be considered.

○   **What is the *most common* cause of airway obstruction in an unconscious patient?**

The tongue.

○   **What percentage of PEs are caused by DVTs?**

95%.

○   **What should the nurse suspect with the following: two or more rib fractures in two or more areas and paradoxical chest movement of this area?**

Flail chest.

○   **What is a priority nursing diagnosis for the patient with a flail chest?**

Impaired gas exchange related to pain.

○   **What is a priority nursing diagnosis for the patient with an acute asthma attack?**

Ineffective airway clearance (related) to impaired airway resistance and inflamed lung tissue (secondary) to bronchospasm, as evidenced by increased secretions, inability to breathe, and feelings of impending doom.

○   **What is a priority nursing diagnosis for the patient with acute respiratory distress syndrome (ARDS)?**

Impaired gas exchange.

○   **A pulmonary embolus (PE) is suspected. What medical diagnostic test is the most accurate in confirming this?**

Pulmonary angiogram. However, this is not the usual test performed. Most workups will include a d-dimer blood test, and if this is positive, or if clinical suspicion is high, then a CT scan of the chest or a V-Q scan (a lung ventilation-perfusion nuclear test) may be done to diagnose a PE. The pulmonary angiogram is done in questionable cases to verify the diagnosis in rare cases. Doppler ultrasound of the extremities may be indicated in some patients to r/o DVT (deep venous thrombophlebitis).

○   **What should be the nurse's initial treatment of a patient with a suspected pulmonary emboli?**

Administer oxygen. Remember—airway, breathing, circulation. Establish one or two IVs, and give IV fluid boluses as indicated.

○   **What are the risk factors associated with pulmonary embolus?**

History of a PE in the past, DVT, obesity, recent surgery, birth control pills, trauma, pregnancy, smoking, and immobility such as a recent long car or airplane trip. Some hormone replacement therapy (HRT) meds have also been known to cause thrombus formation with subsequent emboli.

○   **A 50-year-old female is diagnosed with a moderate PE and has stable vital signs at this time. What anticoagulation options are available and why are they given?**

This patient needs to have her blood thinned by heparin, Lovenox (enoxaparin), or Coumadin. These are given to inhibit further clot formation/emboli development, and allow the body to better resorb the clot or DVT. When using heparin the PTT (partial thromboplastin time) should be between 1.5 and 2 times the control (60–70 seconds). When using coumadin (warfarin), the PT (prothrombin time) should be maintained between 1.5 and 2 times the control (11–12 seconds) or the INR (international normalized ratio) should be between 2 and 3. Once the PT is therapeutic, then the heparin or Lovenox can be discontinued.

○   **A trauma victim presents with shock, decreased breath sounds, dyspnea, and a mediastinal shift. What should you suspect?**

Hemothorax or tension pneumothorax. A FAST ultrasound scan will identify pleural fluid and other things. Placement of a chest tube will be diagnostic and possibly therapeutic. If a tension pneumothorax is suspected, then immediate needle thoracostomy is indicated.

○   **A patient with a hemothorax has a chest tube inserted, massive blood loss in the drainage chamber and the patient begins to decompensate. What procedure should the nurse anticipate?**

Emergency thoracotomy. The bleeding from the large vessels must be clamped or controlled, otherwise the patient will die.

○   **What findings would be expected in the patient exhibiting hyperventilation?**

Increased respiratory rate, anxiety, diaphoresis, diffuse chest pain, jaw pain, and carpopedal spasms.

○   **A patient being treated for an acute asthma attack has been assessed and placed on oxygen. What should be the next intervention?**

Administration of nebulized bronchodilators such as albuterol and ipratropium (Atrovent), usually via nebulizer. Steroids should be given in nearly all cases unless contraindicated. If critically ill, then consider epinephrine, heliox, and possibly intubated in rare circumstances. An IV should also be initiated to give intravenous medications, as well as a cardiac monitor to assess rhythm.

○   **The above patient has received two nebulizer treatments without improvement and becomes agitated. The pulse oximeter has dropped to 80. What possible intervention should the nurse prepare for?**

Intubation. This should be avoided if possible, unless absolutely necessary, due to the worse outcome. Rapid sequence intubation should possibly include use of intravenous ketamine for sedation as it also acts as a bronchodilator.

○   **During the initial treatment of a client with a pulmonary contusion, how should fluid therapy be managed?**

If the patient is hemodynamically stable, fluids should be restricted. Fluid overload can lead to complications such as ARDS and hypoxia.

○   **What is the mortality rate of ARDS?**

Over 50% of patients with ARDS die, usually due to multisystem failure.

○   **What are the risk factors for ARDS?**

Head injury, drug overdose, aspiration pneumonia, hemorrhagic shock, massive blood transfusions, transfusion reactions, near-drowning, pulmonary contusion, smoke inhalation, sepsis, and trauma.

○ **What is atelectasis?**

The partial or total collapse of the functioning alveoli, caused by infection, airway obstruction, COPD, ascites, obesity, smoking, pain, drug use, tumor, pneumothorax, lung compression from large hemothorax, and is common postoperatively for abdomen and thoracic surgery.

○ **What are the signs and symptoms of a tension pneumothorax?**

Cyanosis, hypotension, tachycardia, asymmetrical lung expansion, distended neck veins, chest pain, respiratory distress, and subcutaneous emphysema. Rarely tracheal deviation away from the collapsed lung is noted—this is a late sign. Decreased or absent breath sounds on the affected side.

○ **What is the initial step or test that should be done if a tension pneumothorax is suspected and the patient is critically ill ... get a chest x-ray to confirm or go ahead with needle decompression of the suspected tension pneumothorax?**

If the patient is hypotensive with altered mental status and a tension pneumothorax is suspected clinically, then an emergent chest decompression should immediately be performed prior to any chest x-ray. Some experts feel that a chest x-ray that shows a tension pneumothorax is a mistake ... it should have been treated prior.

○ **Describe the pathophysiology behind a tension pneumothorax:**

Trauma or spontaneous collapse of the lung on one side occurs, and subsequent ventilations of the bag-valve-mask or endotracheal tube cause positive pressure air to leak and escape from the lung into the pleural cavity (intrathoracic), where the air becomes trapped. Additional air causes the pressure to increase, causing increased shifting of the mediastinum which compromises the other lung and also causes the softer large blood veins (such as vena cava) to collapse or kink and block blood flow to the heart. If no blood flow goes into the heart, then no blood goes out, and shock and eventual death may occur.

○ **What is COPD and causes it?**

COPD is chronic obstructive pulmonary disease and is a group of disorders that block the normal flow of air through the lungs, thus trapping air in the alveoli. This includes chronic bronchitis, asthma, and emphysema. The causes primarily are lung irritants such as smoking, dust, and pollen, and some are genetically related.

○ **Which vaccinations are important for COPD patients to get routinely?**

A yearly influenza vaccine and pneumococcal vaccine every 5-10 years to reduce the risk of these infections.

○ **What is emphysema?**

A type of COPD disease of the lung parenchyma where changes and damage in the alveolar wall results in enlarged alveoli distal to the nonrespiratory bronchioles, and is usually associated with continued smoking, second-hand smoke, and alph1-antitrypsin deficiency.

○ **What are the causes of hemothorax?**

Hemothorax is blood in the pleural cavity, and results from chest trauma (penetrating and blunt), lacerated liver, perforated diaphragm, rib fractures, cancer, and other causes.

○ **What are the four major types of malignant tumors that involve the lungs?**

Squamous cell carcinoma, small cell and large cell carcinoma, and adenocarcinoma.

○   **Many lung cancers are metastatic from cancer elsewhere (40%). Name four areas or organs that commonly spread to the lungs.**

Breast, GI, prostate, and renal cancers metastasize to the lung commonly.

○   **What is the most aggressive lung cancer that rapidly spreads but responds to chemotherapy?**

Small cell carcinoma of the lungs.

○   **What is a pleural effusion?**

An accumulation of fluid in the pleural space, which occurs secondary to other disease states. This fluid may contain many leukocytes and pus (empyema), blood (hemothorax), or chyle (chylothorax, from lymphatic fluid leakage). Thoracentesis may be needed for diagnosis and treatment.

○   **What is pulmonary edema and what can cause it?**

The collection of fluid in the extravascular tissues of the lungs, caused by fluid overload, left-sided heart failure, mitral stenosis, ARDS, MI, PE, neurogenic (brain intracranial hemorrhage/bleed or tumor), aspiration, inhalation of toxins, and other causes.

○   **A 68-year old male is admitted with severe CHF and pulmonary edema. A mnemonic for use of medications/treatment is "LMNOP." Name the meds or treatment.**

LMNOP stands for Lasix, Morphine, Nitrates, Oxygen, and if severe, P for pass the endotracheal tube (intubation).

CHAPTER 5 **Gastrointestinal Pearls**

○ **After a week, an ill-appearing patient says her sore throat is much worse and she complains of spiking fevers and central chest burning. What is your concern?**

Retro- or parapharyngeal abscess with extension to the mediastinum.

○ **A 40-year old smoker describes acute, crescendo substernal chest tightness going to his back, unrelieved by antacids. An ECG shows mild nonspecific ST-T changes, and his pain changes from 6/10 to 0/10 approximately 10 minutes after a nitroglycerin tablet. Is this angina?**

Maybe, though the delayed response to nitrates characterizes "esophageal colic" caused by segmental esophageal spasm, often triggered by reflux. Patients with atypical chest pain and an abnormal ECG will likely need to be admitted overnight to rule out an MI vs other etiology.

○ **A patient with an "acid stomach" develops melena and vomits bright red blood. Is esophagitis a likely cause?**

No. Capillary bleeding rarely causes impressive acute blood loss. Arterial bleeding (from a complicated ulcer, foreign body, or Mallory-Weiss tear) or variceal bleeding is much more likely.

○ **A cirrhotic patient vomits bright red blood. He has a systolic blood pressure of 90 mm Hg. After an aggressive fluid resuscitation, 4 units of PRBC and gastric lavage, his pressure is 90 mm Hg. What blood product should also be administered?**

Transfuse fresh frozen plasma to aid in restoring the clotting mechanism.

○ **Recurrent pneumonias, especially in the right middle lobe or the superior segments of the bilateral upper lobes, suggests what syndrome?**

Aspiration, associated with motor diseases and gastroesophageal reflux.

○ **List four contraindications to introduction of a nasogastric tube.**

(1) Suspected esophageal laceration or perforation.

(2) Near obstruction due to stricture.

(3) Esophageal foreign body.

(4) Severe head trauma with rhinorrhea (basilar skull fracture).

○ **Repeated violent bouts of vomiting can result in both Mallory-Weiss tears and Boerhaave syndrome. Differentiate the two.**

Mallory-Weiss tears involve the submucosa and mucosa, typically in the right posterolateral wall of the GE junction.
Boerhaave is a full-thickness tear or rupture, usually in the unsupported left posterolateral wall of the abdominal esophagus.

○ **After a high-speed MVA, an unrestrained driver develops abdominal and chest pain radiating to the neck. You review with the physician the chest x-ray, which shows left pleural fluid. What gastroesophageal catastrophe might have occurred?**

Impact against a steering wheel can result in Boerhaave's syndrome—ruptured esophagus with perforation and mediastinitis.

○ **When is removing a button battery lodged in the esophagus indicated?**

Battery ingestion always calls for removal because of its toxic nature. If not removed, it can cause esophageal erosion, perforation, and occasionally erode into the nearby aorta causing exsanguinating hemorrhage.

○ **Most objects, even sharp ones, pass through the GI tract without incident. What objects should be removed?**

Any object that obstructs or perforates, that is >5 cm long and >2 cm wide (won't make it past the GE junction), or is toxic (batteries) should be removed, either endoscopically or surgically. Sharp or pointed objects (sewing needles and razor blades) should be removed if they haven't passed the pylorus.

○ **Name two endocrine problems that cause peptic ulcer.**

Zollinger-Ellison syndrome and hyperparathyroidism (hypercalcemia).

○ **In a patient with early satiety and ulcer symptoms, what clinical finding essentially rules out a gastric outlet obstruction?**

Bilious vomitus.

○ **Burning epigastric pain shooting to the back, hypovolemic shock, and a high amylase suggests . . .**

Posterior perforation of a duodenal ulcer.

○ **Enteric coated potassium tablets, typhoid, tuberculosis, tumors, and strangulated hernia may cause what rare process?**

Nontraumatic small-bowel perforation.

○ **What is the *most common* cause of lower GI perforation?**

Diverticulitis, followed by tumor, colitis, foreign bodies, and instrumentation.

○ **A pregnant woman with right upper quadrant pain should be assumed to have what intra-abdominal pathology until proven otherwise?**

Acute appendicitis. In pregnancy, the appendix is shifted upwards, causing a higher localization of pain with appendicitis.

○ **Rovsing's, psoas, and obturator signs can all indicate an inflamed posterior appendix. Please describe these signs.**

Rovsing's sign—right lower quadrant pain when the left lower quadrant is palpated.

Psoas sign—right lower quadrant pain on right thigh extension.

Obturator sign—right lower quadrant pain on internal rotation of the flexed right thigh.

○ **What is the *most common* cause of small bowel obstruction?**

Adhesions, mostly due to prior surgery with scar tissue causing adhesion of intestines together, along with other organs and peritoneal surfaces.

○ **What are the *most common* causes of colonic obstruction?**

Cancer is the most common cause, then diverticulitis, followed by volvulus.

○ **List three classes of drugs that cause pseudo-obstruction (distention of intestines from medications, not a surgical obstruction):**

Anticholinergics, antiparkinsonian drugs, and tricyclic antidepressants.

○ **A young man with atraumatic chronic back pain, eye trouble, and painful red lumps on his shins develops *bloody diarrhea*. What is the point of this question?**

To remind you of extraintestinal manifestations of inflammatory bowel disease, such as ankylosing spondylitis, uveitis, and erythema nodosum, not to mention *kidney stones*.

○ **A patient with chronic, occasionally bloody diarrhea develops severe diarrhea and abdominal pain with marked distention. What syndrome does this describe?**

Toxic megacolon, a life-threatening complication of ulcerative colitis.

○ **A patient with new diarrhea and abdominal pain tells you she took antibiotics for sinusitis 2 weeks ago. What syndrome could she have developed?**

Pseudomembranous colitis, which is usually caused when a patient takes antibiotics, causing the normal intestinal bacteria to die, with abnormal bacterial overgrowth including *Clostridium difficile,* a gram-positive, spore-forming, anaerobic bacillus, which is present in almost all of these cases. Medicines mostly involved include clindamycin, lincomycin, ampicillin, or cephalosporin, but any antimicrobial agent (including antifungal, antiviral, and metronidazole) could incite the disease, regardless of the amount administered or the route of administration. It is diagnosed by a *C. difficile* stool antigen test or by colonoscopy.

○ **What's the treatment for pseudomembranous colitis?**

For most fairly healthy patients, use oral metronidazole, 500 mg TID × 10 days. For pregnant patients or more seriously ill patients, use oral vancomycin 125 mg qid × 10 days.

○ **Is diverticulitis the likely diagnosis in a patient with low abdominal pain and bright red blood per rectum?**

No. Typically diverticul*osis* bleeds, while diverticu*litis* doesn't. Diverticulosis bleeding is typically painless.

○ **Abdominal pain in a gray-haired patient should always suggest_____, until proven otherwise.**

Mesenteric ischemia.

○ **Which is more sensitive for locating the source of GI bleeding, a radioactive Tc-labeled red cell scan or angiography?**

A bleeding scan can find a site bleeding at a rate as low as 0.12 ml/min, while angiography requires rapid bleeding (greater than 0.5 ml/min).

○ **In addition to conjugated hyperbilirubinemia, what liver function abnormalities suggest biliary tract disease?**

Elevated alkaline phosphatase out of proportion to transaminases. This enzyme is abnormally high when gallstones cause obstruction of the biliary tract system with resultant cholecystitis or other biliary tract infection.

○ **A cirrhotic presents with weakness and edema. What electrolyte imbalances might be present?**

Hyponatremia (dilutional or diuretic-induced), hypokalemia (from GI losses, secondary hyperaldosteronism, or diuretics), and hypomagnesemia.

○ **The best diuretic choice for most cirrhotics with ascites?**

Potassium-sparing agents (treat the hyperaldosterone state specifically).

○ **A confused cirrhotic presents to you. She is afebrile and has asterixis. What should your exam consist of as you look for the precipitant of hepatic encephalopathy?**

Assess her mental status and search for localizing neurologic signs (occult head injury); look for dry mucous membranes and a low jugular venous pressure (hypovolemia and azotemia); check a stool guaiac (GI bleeding).

○ **Aside from fixing the above, what therapy is useful?**

Lactulose, which produces an acidic diarrhea that traps nitrogenous wastes in the gut.

○ **The *most common* organism responsible for spontaneous bacterial peritonitis (SBP)?**

E. coli, followed by *S. pneumoniae*.

○ **A nondrinker presents with acute pancreatitis. What conditions may underlie this acute process?**

Biliary tract disease, trauma (blunt or penetrating), ulcers (posterior penetrating duodenal ulcer), diabetes (ketoacidosis), cancer, and hypertriglyceridemia.

○ **Distinguish anal chancres and herpetic ulcers.**

Anal chancres of primary syphilis are *painful*, symmetric, indurated, and diagnosed by dark-field microscopy. Herpes simplex produces perianal paresthesias and pruritus, followed by red-haloed vesicles and apthous ulcers (ruptured vesicles); a Tzanck smear is diagnostic. Both cause painful inguinal adenopathy.

○ **What stool studies are crucial in evaluating acute diarrhea?**

Statistically speaking, acute diarrhea is so common and typically self-limited that *most cases need no testing*, just oral rehydration. The exception is patients who have complications, or in whom the diarrhea lasts longer than 4 days and fever is present. In sick patients or those at risk for complications (at the extremes of age, recently hospitalized, immunocompromised), *enteroinvasive infection should be ruled out* with a stool guaiac and test for fecal leukocytes (Gram or methylene blue stains are comparable).

○ **The *most common* cause of bacterial diarrhea?**

E. coli (enteroinvasive, enteropathogenic, enterotoxigenic).

○ **A former IV drug user with sickle-cell disease and a history of splenectomy presents with unremitting fever, crampy abdominal pain, and meningismus after recently acquiring a pet turtle. He has no diarrhea. What bacteria may be the culprit?**

Salmonella typhi, the causative agent of typhoid fever. The attack rate is remarkably high in patients with HIV, in asplenic patients, and in those with sickle cell disease. Rose spots occur in 10–20%; relative bradycardia in the face of a high fever, and a low or normal WBC with a pronounced left shift are suggestive findings.

○ **Match the diarrheal syndrome with the culprit:**

(1) *Aeromonas hydrophila*	— Diarrhea on the way to the car after eating fried rice at a Chinese buffet.
(2) *Bacillus cereus*	— Diarrhea followed by thigh myalgias, perioral dysesthesias, and pruritus.
(3) Campylobacter	— Profuse, foul-smelling diarrhea with bloating and cramps after a fishing trip.
(4) *Clostridium difficile*	— Bloody diarrhea and fever in a child.
(5) *Clostridium perfringens*	— Acute dysentery, fever, and pseudoappendicitis after getting a new puppy.
(6) *Vibrio parahemolyticus*	— Rice water diarrhea without fever or constitutional symptoms.
(7) *Staph Aureus*	— Diarrhea from raw seafood.
(8) Yersinia	— Diarrhea from contaminated meat; no nausea or vomiting.
(9) Giardia	— Diarrhea from antibiotic-associated enterocolitis.
(10) Ciguatera toxin	— Diarrhea (enterocolitis) associated with either antibiotics *or* food.

Answers: 2, 10, 9, 3, 8, 1, 6, 5, 4, 7.

Diarrhea on the way to the car after eating fried rice at a Chinese buffet—*Bacillus cereus*; treatment is symptomatic.

Diarrhea followed by thigh myalgias, perioral dysesthesias, and pruritus—Ciguatera toxin; no treatment.

Profuse, foul-smelling diarrhea with bloating and cramps after a fishing trip—Giardia; quinacrine or metronidazole.

Bloody diarrhea and fever in a child—Campylobacter; erythromycin; doxycycline or fluoroquinolone in adults.

Acute dysentery, fever and pseudoappendicitis—Yersinia; optimal tx unknown, chloramphenicol, tetracycline, TMP/SMX.

Rice water diarrhea without fever or constitutional symptoms—*Aeromonas hydrophilia* with sx due to enterotoxin; tx primarily symptomatic.

Diarrhea from raw seafood—*Vibrio parahemolyticus*; treat symptoms.

Diarrhea from contaminated meat; no nausea or vomiting—*Clostridium perfringens*; usually no therapy, rarely antitoxin antibodies.

Diarrhea from antibiotic-associated enterocolitis—*Clostridium difficile*; vancomycin or metronidazole.

Diarrhea (enterocolitis) associated with either antibiotics or food—*Staph aureus*; treat symptoms.

○ **What are the symptoms most commonly associated with neuromuscular associated dysphagia?**

Nasopharyngeal regurgitation and hoarseness.

○ **The *most common* causes of dysphagia in the elderly population include:**

Hiatal hernia, reflux esophagitis, webs/rings, and cancer.

○ **The *most common* symptom of esophageal disease is?**

Pyrosis: heartburn.

○ **What are the classical features that distinguish chest pain of esophageal origin from cardiac ischemia?**

There are no classical clinical features that distinguish between these two entities. Exertional pain and palliation with rest or NTG occur in both groups. Pain relief in the GI group usually takes 7–10 minutes while ischemic pain usually responds in 2–3 minutes. However, most patients will need to be observed overnight in the hospital with serial ECG and cardiac enzymes to rule out acute coronary syndromes versus other diagnoses.

○ **What medical conditions are associated with an increase incidence of peptic ulcer disease (PUD)?**

COPD, cirrhosis, and chronic renal failure.

○ **What type of patients are at risk for gallbladder perforation?**

Elderly, diabetics and those with recurrent cholecystitis.

○ **What is a positive Murphy's sign?**

Pain that is worsened with abdomen palpation of the right upper quadrant during inspiration, which is often a finding in patients with cholecystitis (gallbladder infection).

○ **What is cirrhosis?**

A chronic, progressive disease that causes extensive degeneration and destruction of the liver; there are multiple types and causes of cirrhosis.

○ **A 55-year-old male who has a history of chronic alcohol abuse and cirrhosis, is admitted after vomiting blood. Soon after admission, he is found weak, pale, diaphoretic, and has vomited a large amount of bright red blood. Describe treatment options for bleeding esophageal varices.**

Consider blood transfusion, transfer to an ICU, give vasopressin, beta-adrenergic blocker; endoscopic sclerosis, possibly inserting a Sengstaken-Blakemore tube or various surgical shunts. Surgery may be indicated for severe, rare cases.

○ **What are the causes of acute pancreatitis?**

Alcohol abuse, infection, drug ingestion/toxicity, trauma, smoking, obstruction of the biliary tract or pancreatic duct, and other etiologies are causes of acute pancreatitis.

○ **What are the indications for the surgical removal of a GI foreign body?**

GI obstruction; GI perforation; toxic properties of the material, length, size, and shape that will prevent the object from passing safely.

○ **What size objects rarely pass the stomach?**

Objects longer than 5 cm and wider than 2 cm.

○ **What are the *most common* causes of nontraumatic perforations of the lower GI tract?**

Diverticulitis, carcinoma, colitis, foreign bodies, barium enemas, and endoscopy.

○ **The hallmark of a perforated viscus is?**

Abdominal pain.

○ **What is the bacteria that has been found inside the stomach of patients with peptic ulcer disease?**

H. pylori

○ **A 46-year-old male is admitted with peptic ulcer disease. Name the causes of PUD and treatment.**

Erosion of the lining cells of the stomach or duodenum is caused by NSAIDS and *H. pylori*, and patients are at increased risk when they smoke, drink alcohol, use caffeine, or are stressed at work or home. Treatment may include histamine blockers (cimetidine, ranitidine, famotidine, nizatidine) to decrease gastric acid production; antacids may be given orally to neutralize stomach acid; PPIs (proton pump inhibitors such as lansoprazole or omeprazole) are increasingly used to decrease acid production; sucralfate is given orally to form a protective barrier over an ulcer's surface; cessation of smoking, drinking, caffeine, and decreasing stress are also helpful. In severe or resistant cases of peptic ulcer disease, endoscopy or surgery may be required.

○ **What are the more common processes that mimic acute appendicitis?**

Mesenteric lymphadenitis, PID, mittleshmertz, gastroenteritis, and Crohn's disease.

○ **What are the most frequent symptoms of acute appendicitis?**

Anorexia and pain. The classical presentation: anorexia, periumbilical pain with progression toward the RLQ, with constant RLQ pain. This presentation occurs in only 60% of cases.

○ **What clinical maneuvers may aid in the diagnosis of acute appendicitis?**

The psoas sign and the obturator sign may aid in the diagnosis of an inflamed posteriorly located appendix.

○ **What percentage of acute appendicitis cases has an elevated WBC count?**

An elevated leukocyte count and an elevated absolute neutrophil count are present in 86% and 89%, respectively.

○ **A patient presents with palmar erythema, spider angiomas, testicular atrophy, and asterixis. What is the most likely cause?**

This patient has cirrhosis.

○ **What are some other findings observed in a patient with cirrhosis?**

Hematemesis, encephalopathy, hepatomegaly, splenomegaly, jaundice, caput medusa, ascites, and gynecomastia may also occur.

○ **Which is the *most common* form of acute diarrhea?**

Viral diarrhea. It is generally self-limited, lasting only 1–3 days.

○ **What is the most probable cause of diarrhea that develops within 12 hours of a meal?**

An ingested preformed toxin, such as staphylococcal food poisoning from food that is left out of the refrigerator too long, or old left-over foods.

○   **When does traveler's diarrhea typically occur?**

3–7 days after arrival in a foreign land.

○   **What is the definition of chronic diarrhea?**

The passage of greater than 200 g of loose stool per day for over 3 weeks.

○   **What syndrome is indicated by crampy abdominal pain and mucus-filled stool?**

Irritable bowel syndrome. Patients are afebrile and often improve after passing flatus.

○   **What layers of the bowel are involved in regional ileitis (Crohn's disease) and ulcerative colitis?**

All layers of the bowel in various areas (skip areas) of the bowel at the same time are involved in regional ileitis (Crohn's). Only the mucosal and submucosal layers are involved, in a continuous diffuse manner in ulcerative colitis.

○   **Epigastric pain that radiates to the back and is relieved, to some extent, by sitting up is indicative of what disease?**

Pancreatitis.

○   **What is the *most common* gastrointestinal complaint in AIDS patients?**

Diarrhea. Hepatomegaly and hepatitis are also typical. Cryptosporidium and Isospora are common causes of prolonged watery diarrhea.

○   **In the elderly, what is a common side effect of verapamil?**

Constipation.

○   **What is the *most common* cause of abdominal pain in the elderly?**

Constipation.

○   **How is jaundice diagnosed in an African American patient?**

Darkly pigmented patients often have subconjunctival fat that results in yellowing the sclera. In patients where icterus is suspected, it is imperative to examine the edges of the cornea and the posterior hard palate.

○   **How does pallor appear in an African American patient?**

The skin is yellow/brown or gray due to the loss of the underlying red tones. The conjunctiva will appear pale.

○   **What is the *most common* cause of a paralytic ileus?**

Surgery.

○   **How is hepatitis A transmitted?**

By the oral fecal route. No carrier state exists. A common way to acquire this infection is to eat food (fruit, beverages with ice, etc.) that is contaminated by a worker who does not wash their hands well.

○ **What is a potential side effect of the use of Kayexalate?**

Kayexalate exchanges sodium for K+. As a result, sodium overload and CHF may occur.

○ **What is the danger of taking Isoniazid (INH) and drinking alcohol on a frequent basis?**

Isoniazid related hepatitis.

○ **What symptoms would you expect to find in a patient who has a perforated duodenal ulcer?**

Abdominal rigidity and tenderness.

○ **What are some of the common symptoms associated with pancreatitis?**

Intense midepigastric abdominal pain radiating to the back with nausea and vomiting.

○ **What is the preferred way to determine if a nasogastric tube has been correctly inserted?**

Apply suction to the tube and observe for the return of stomach contents, and instill air into the tube while auscultating over the epigastric area.

○ **What stool color indicates that a patient may have bleeding in the upper GI tract?**

Black. This color may be found in patients taking iron supplements, pepto-bismal, and other medications.

○ **A medsurg nurse is caring for a patient with active upper-GI bleeding, and the patient is hungry soon after admission. What is the appropriate diet for the patient during the first 24 hours after admission?**

Nothing by mouth. Bleeding and any shock must be controlled before giving anything orally. A liquid diet is given when able to be tolerated by the patient. Cool fluids should be used when restarting an oral diet.

○ **What lab value would be elevated in a patient with pancreatitis?**

Serum amylase and lipase.

○ **When assessing bowel sounds, why should you auscultate the abdomen before palpation?**

Palpating the abdomen first could affect bowel sounds.

○ **How long should you listen in each quadrant to confirm the absence of bowel sounds?**

5 minutes. However few medical professionals will wait that long. An absence of any bowel sounds over a 20–30 second time span indicates significant slowing of borborygmi sounds (the noise that intestines make).

○ **What type of solution should be used to irrigate a nasogastric tube and why?**

Normal saline. Usage of hypotonic or hypertonic solutions could cause electrolyte imbalances.

○ **Why should you be concerned if a patient with a nasogastric tube complains of nausea, vomiting, and abdominal distention?**

These are the symptoms that the nasogastric tube was likely placed to prevent. It could mean the nasogastric tube is not functioning properly. If the NG tube is causing gagging and nausea due to stimulation of the oropharynx, then consider giving lidocaine or benzocaine spray to the throat to make the patient more comfortable. Need to reassess placement (via pH, aspiration, x-ray, etc.) and then flush to try to restart appropriate suction.

○ **What is the major cause of acute pancreatitis in the United States?**

Alcoholism.

○ **What is the pathophysiology of pancreatitis?**

Stimulation of pancreatic enzymes causes an autodigestive process of the pancreas to occur.

○ **What is the purpose of administering aluminum hydroxide (Amphojel) to a patient?**

It is an antacid used in the treatment of gastritis or an ulcer. It may also be used in patients with kidney disease to help bind the excess phosphate in the intestines and decrease the phosphate level.

○ **What is the primary purpose of maintaining an IV in a patient with a nasogastric tube?**

To optimize fluid and electrolyte balance, and maintenance of fluid replacement.

○ **What is the primary indication for the use of prochlorperazine (Compazine)?**

It is used as an antiemetic. Although rare, monitor for dystonic reactions (thickened tongue speech and control problems, neck muscle spasm, and a feeling of anxiety and agitation). If noted, then treat with diphenhydramine.

○ **What should be checked when gastric distention is noted in a patient with a nasogastric tube?**

Check the wall suction or other device to ensure it is working properly, ensure the patency of the tube and connections and the tube's placement. Gastric fluid pH may be checked to conform proper placement.

○ **Why does a patient with cholecystitis exhibit nausea, vomiting, and abdominal discomfort after eating a high fat meal?**

The digestion of fats is impaired due to the insufficient flow of bile from the gallbladder.

○ **What is the function of ranitidine (Zantac)?**

Decrease gastric acid secretion by blocking the H2 receptor in the stomach.

○ **What is the function of omeprazole and lansoprazole?**

These are PPI (proton pump inhibitors) which suppress acid production by halting the mechanism that pumps acid into the stomach.

○ **What electrolyte imbalance is a complication of pancreatitis?**

Hypocalcemia.

○ **What symptoms would you expect to find in a patient with a hiatal hernia?**

Heartburn is the most common complaint, with regurgitation and dysphagia also present.

○ **What is the purpose of metoclopramide hydrochloride (Reglan) in the treatment of a hiatal hernia?**

It increases sphincter tone and promotes gastric emptying.

○ **A patient with a potential surgical abdomen complains of abdominal pain upon admission but the physician refuses to administer pain medication until his/her abdomen is assessed. What is the reason for this?**

Some physicians mistakenly believe that narcotics may mask symptoms of pain, which is often used as an indication of the severity of the patient's condition. Multiple studies have shown that moderate medication doses do not interfere with accurate diagnoses. Therefore, pain medications should not be withheld in patients with severe pain.

○ **What is the purpose of lactulose (Chronulac) administration in cirrhosis?**

It decreases ammonia formation in the intestine by increasing intestinal motility and causing diarrhea.

○ **A physician orders sodium polystyrene sulfonate (Kayexalate). What would be the most likely reason for administering this drug?**

To help lower the patient's high serum potassium level.

○ **What is the best position for an unconscious patient undergoing a gastric lavage?**

Lateral position with head of the bed tilted downward, or semiprone position.

○ **What type of ulcer is characterized by pain 2 hours after eating, and is relieved by eating more food, drinking milk, or taking an antacid?**

Duodenal ulcer.

○ **What type of ulcer is characterized by pain during or shortly after eating a meal?**

Gastric ulcer.

○ **What are the signs and symptoms of a perforated peptic ulcer?**

Sudden severe upper abdominal pain, vomiting, and a tender rigid abdomen.

○ **What is the name of the bacteria that when found in the stomach is associated with a much higher rate of peptic ulcer disease**

H. pylori is the name of the bacteria.

○ **What is Cullen's sign?**

A bluish discoloration around the umbilicus of a postoperative patient or a patient with retroperitoneal bleeding (such as from a ruptured AAA or trauma).

○ **What does Cullen's sign indicate?**

Intra-abdominal or peritoneal bleeding.

○   **What are the signs and symptoms of a small bowel obstruction?**

Decreased bowel sounds, abdominal distention, decreased flatus, and projectile vomiting.

○   **What are the signs and symptoms of acute pancreatitis?**

Low grade fever, tachycardia, hypotension, discolored flank (Grey Turner's sign), vomiting, and epigastric pain.

○   **If a client has ascites from chronic liver disease, what position should help with respiration?**

The semi-Fowler's position.

○   **What is the most sensitive test for liver dysfunction?**

Prothrombin time.

○   **What is the most fatal complication of severe acute pancreatitis?**

Hypovolemia.

○   **Where on the body does jaundice first manifest?**

The sclera.

○   **What is the first symptom of pancreatitis?**

A constant epigastric pain that radiates to the back.

○   **What is obstipation?**

Extreme intractable constipation caused by an intestinal obstruction.

○   **What is a reducible hernia?**

A protruding mass that can be pushed and placed back into the abdomen.

○   **What is the *most common* symptom of hepatitis A?**

Anorexia.

○   **What does a positive Murphy's sign indicate?**

Cholecystitis.

○   **What is normal serum amylase level?**

25–125 U/l.

○   **What is an absolute contraindication to a peritoneal lavage?**

Distended bladder.

○   **What is the primary nursing diagnosis in the patient with a bowel obstruction?**

Fluid volume deficit.

○ **What is the primary nursing diagnosis for the patient who has been vomiting frequently and has developed metabolic alkalosis?**

Fluid and electrolyte imbalance.

○ **What electrolyte is in danger of being depleted with prolonged vomiting?**

Potassium.

○ **What nursing intervention would be indicated for the patient admitted to the ER with an acute GI bleed?**

Start two large bore IVs, insert a nasogastric tube (NGT), draw blood for CBC, and Type and Crossmatch.

○ **A patient has been admitted to the hospital after ingesting a corrosive substance. In addition to concerns and treatment of the GI tract, what should the nurse monitor?**

Airway status. Chemical burns to the back of the throat could cause an airway obstruction. Esophageal perforation can occur, or aspiration may be present.

○ **The patient with abdominal pain, fever, nausea, and vomiting is thirsty and is waiting to be seen by the doctor. You suspect the flu and give the patient clear liquids. The doctor walks in and gives you an angry look. Why?**

The patient could have a surgical abdomen. Any undiagnosed abdominal pain should remain NPO until cleared by a physician.

○ **The nurse accesses the client and notes bright red GI bleeding per rectum. Is this an upper or lower GI bleed?**

Can't determine. Rapid upper GI bleeding that passes through the GI tract quickly can produce the same symptoms. Some physicians will consider briefly placing a NG tube and aspirating this to see if there is any blood leaking into the stomach. Most cases of bright red blood per rectum are from a lower GI bleed source.

○ **The EMTs arrive with a patient with a known history of alcohol abuse. He had been vomiting bright red blood profusely and is now unconscious. Vitals show a low blood pressure, increased pulse rate, and increased respirations. A new intern shouts, "Give vitamin K, draw labs, get an accucheck, insert an IV, insert an NGT, insert a Foley, call the blood bank!" What should you do first?**

Protect yourself and your staff first, by putting on appropriate PPE (personal protective equipment) which includes full universal precautions including protective goggles, mask, gloves, gown, and head and shoe protection. Assume every patient has a deadly disease that may be transmitted. Then remember the ABC's. This patient is most likely intoxicated, vomiting, and he is unconscious with a low BP. Protect the airway. Establish a safety net of IV, oxygen, monitor, and pulse oximetry. Then pursue and/or delegate other actions

○ **What is the priority nursing diagnosis in the client with intussusception?**

Altered tissue perfusion. Fluid volume deficit may occur secondary to the altered tissue perfusion.

○ **While assisting the physician with the insertion of a Sengstaken-Blackmore tube, the patient suddenly develops severe respiratory distress. What intervention should be done immediately?**

The tube could be causing an obstruction. Remove the tube.

○ **What is an important part of nursing care for the patient with a Sengstaken-Blackmore tube?**

Mouth care and oral suctioning. The patient cannot swallow oral secretions. Monitor for rebleeding and a deterioration of vital signs.

○ **A patient arrives with a knife sticking out of his abdomen and he is hemodynamically unstable. The physician wants a DPL (diagnostic peritoneal lavage). Why should you question this order?**

Obvious abdominal trauma and unstable. A DPL would only waste time. It serves no diagnostic purpose and wastes time... if the patient is going to surgery or getting a CT scan then it has no significant purpose. This patient needs to get to the OR fast.

○ **What symptoms would you suspect in the patient with peritonitis?**

Guarding pain, decreased bowel sounds, nausea, vomiting, and possible fever.

○ **Irritants *inside* the bowel will cause what type of bowel sounds?**

Hyperactive. Irritants outside of the bowel will likely result in hypoactive bowel sounds.

○ **The trauma patient complains of left shoulder pain but no injury is found to the area. What should the nurse suspect?**

Bleeding in the abdomen causing diaphragmatic irritation.

○ **While assessing the trauma patient, you hear bowel sounds in the chest. What should you suspect?**

Diaphragmatic rupture, which is more common on the left side (the liver spreads across the under side of the right diaphragm and is therefore protective against rupture somewhat).

○ **A confused patient's lab values reveal a decreased albumin, increased prothrombin tine, and an increased ammonia level. What should you suspect?**

Liver failure.

CHAPTER 6

Homeostasis, Metabolic and Endocrine Pearls

○ **A 36-year-old female presents with a history of being difficult to arouse in the morning. Her husband says, "After she's had breakfast, she perks right up." What do you suspect?**

Fasting hypoglycemia. Fasting hypoglycemia may reflect serious organic disease. As a consequence, evaluation of this disorder typically requires hospitalization.

○ **What is the principle hormone protecting the human body against hypoglycemia?**

Glucagon.

○ **How is sulfonylurea-induced hypoglycemia treated?**

IV glucose alone may be insufficient. It may require diazoxide 300 mg slow IV over 30 minutes repeated every 4 hours.

○ **What effect does propranolol have on blood sugar in diabetic patients?**

Propranolol may precipitate hypoglycemia. It actually may mask the signs and symptoms of hypoglycemia as a patient may have a low blood sugar and not realize it.

○ **What are the neurologic signs and symptoms of hypoglycemia?**

Hypoglycemia may produce mental and neurologic dysfunction. Common neurologic manifestations may include difficulty in concentrating, confusion, agitation, headache, dizziness, blurred vision, seizures, and loss of consciousness. Other findings may include paresthesias, cranial nerve palsies, transient hemiplegia, diplopia, decerebrate posturing, and clonus. This diagnosis should be ruled out in all patients with altered mental status.

○ **What lab findings are expected with diabetic ketoacidosis?**

Elevated β-hydroxybutyrate, acetoacetate, acetone, and glucose. Ketonuria and glucosuria are present. Serum bicarbonate level, PCO_2 and pH are decreased. Potassium may be initially elevated but falls if the acidosis is corrected. The patient may have a significant potassium depletion and thus, levels should be followed closely and replaced accordingly.

○ **What is the treatment of DKA?**

IV normal saline with aggressive infusion rates (watch carefully in patients with CHF), consider adding potassium to IV fluids when normal renal function is confirmed, with potassium 100–200 mEq in the first 12–24 hours. An

IV insulin drip at 0.1 U/kg should be started. Research studies show debatable benefits of an initial insulin bolus. When starting a drip, the IV insulin should be dripped through the tubing at a high rate prior to hooking to the patient. This will help saturate any binding sites inside the lumen of the plastic tubing. Closely monitor blood glucose levels. Sodium bicarbonate should only rarely be used to treat the acidosis; the patient should correct the acidosis on his own with IV hydration.

○ **What are the complications of bicarbonate therapy in DKA?**

Paradoxical CSF acidosis, cardiac arrhythmias, decreased oxygen delivery to tissue, and fluid and sodium overload.

○ **What sulfonylurea compound most commonly causes hypoglycemia?**

Chlorpropamide.

○ **What are the key features of nonketotic hyperosmolar coma?**

Hyperosmolality, hyperglycemia, and dehydration. Blood sugar should be greater than 800 mg/dL, serum osmolality should be greater than 350 mOsm/kg, and serum ketones should be negative.

○ **What is the treatment of nonketotic hyperosmolar coma?**

Fluids (normal saline), potassium 10–20 mEq/h. Insulin 5–10 U/h and glucose should be added to the IV when the blood sugar drops below 250 mg/dl.

○ **What is the most consistent finding with lactic acidosis?**

Kussmaul's respirations or hyperventilation.

○ **What is the *most common* cause of thyroid storm?**

Infections, typically pulmonary infections, are the most common precipitating events.

○ **What clinical clues might lead you to suspect thyroid storm?**

Eye signs of Graves' disease, a history of hyperthyroidism, widened pulse pressure, and a palpable goiter. Tachycardia, CNS dysfunction, cardiovascular dysfunction, GI system dysfunction, and temperature greater than 37.8°C (100°F).

○ **What is the approximate overall mortality of nonketotic hyperosmolar coma?**

Approximately 50%. Some research indicates that it is between 20–40% with appropriate treatment.

○ **What is the *most common* cause of hypothyroidism?**

Primary thyroid failure. Worldwide the most common cause is insufficient elemental iodine in the diet. In modern countries, the most common etiology of hypothyroidism in adults is autoimmune thyroid disorders (Hashimoto's thyroiditis), and the second most common cause is the use of radioactive iodine or subtotal thyroidectomy in the treatment of Graves' disease.

○ **What is the *most common* cause of secondary adrenal insufficiency and adrenal crisis?**

Iatrogenic adrenal suppression from prolonged steroid use. Rapid withdrawal of steroids may lead to collapse and death.

○ **What are the two primary causes of metabolic alkalosis?**

Loss of hydrogen and chloride from the stomach.
  Overzealous diuresis with loss of hydrogen, potassium, and chloride.

○ **What is central pontine myelinolysis, a.k.a. osmotic demyelination syndrome?**

The complication of brain dehydration following too rapid correction of severe hyponatremia. Correct hyponatremia slowly, less than 12 mEq/d in chronic hyponatremia. A good rule of thumb is to correct the hyponatremia approximately as slowly as it developed.

○ **Which electrolyte imbalances might be present in a cirrhotic patient who presents with weakness and edema?**

Hyponatremia (dilutional or diuretic-induced), hypokalemia (from GI losses, secondary hyperaldosteronism, or diuretics), and hypomagnesemia.

○ **How does hyperglycemia lead to hyponatremia?**

Because glucose stays in the extracellular fluid, hyperglycemia draws water out of the cell into the extracellular fluid. Each 100 mg/dl increase in plasma glucose decreases the serum sodium by 1.6–1.8 mEq/l.

○ **What are the signs and symptoms of hyponatremia?**

Weakness, nausea, anorexia, vomiting, confusion, lethargy, seizures, and coma.

○ **What are the *most common* causes of the hypotonic fluid loss which lead to hypernatremia?**

Diarrhea, vomiting, hyperpyrexia, and excessive sweating.

○ **What are the signs and symptoms of hypernatremia?**

Confusion, muscle irritability, seizures, respiratory paralysis, and coma.

○ **What are the causes of hyperkalemia?**

Acidosis, tissue necrosis, hemolysis, blood transfusions, GI bleed, renal failure, Addison's disease, primary hypoaldosteronism, excess po K+ intake, RTA IV, and medications such as succinylcholine, β-blockers, captopril (Capoten), spironolactone, triamterene, amiloride, and high dose penicillin.

○ **What are the causes of hypocalcemia?**

Shock, sepsis, multiple blood transfusions, hypoparathyroidism, vitamin D deficiency, pancreatitis, hypomagnesemia, alkalosis, fat embolism syndrome, phosphate overload, chronic renal failure, loop diuretics, hypoalbuminemia, tumor lysis syndrome and medication, such as Dilantin, phenobarbital, heparin, theophylline, cimetidine, and gentamicin.

○ **What is the *most common* cause of hyperkalemia?**

Chronic renal failure is the most common cause of "true hyperkalemia."

○ **What are the *most common* causes of hypercalcemia?**

In descending order: malignancy, primary hyperparathyroidism, and thiazide diuretics.

○ **What are the signs and symptoms of hypercalcemia?**

The most common gastrointestinal symptoms are anorexia and constipation. A classic mnemonic can be used to remember them:

Stones: renal calculi.

Bones: osteolysis.

Abdominal groans: peptic ulcer disease and pancreatitis.

Psychic overtones: psychiatric disorders.

○ **What is the initial treatment for hypercalcemia?**

The initial treatment is restoration of the extracellular fluid with 5–10 l of normal saline within 24 hours. After the patient is rehydrated, furosemide (Lasix) in doses of 1–3 mg/kg is usually ordered.

○ **What is the *most common* cause of hyperphosphatemia?**

Acute and chronic renal failure.

○ **What are the signs and symptoms of primary adrenal insufficiency?**

Fatigue, weakness, weight loss, anorexia, hyperpigmentation, nausea, vomiting, abdominal pain, diarrhea, and orthostatic hypotension.

○ **What lab findings are associated with primary adrenal insufficiency (Addison's disease)?**

Hyperkalemia, hyponatremia, hypoglycemia, azotemia (if volume depletion is present), and a mild metabolic acidosis.

○ **What causes acute adrenal crisis?**

It occurs secondary to a major stress, such as surgery, severe injury, myocardial infarction, or any other illness in a patient with primary or secondary adrenal insufficiency. Any patient who is on chronic daily steroids is at higher risk of adrenal crisis.

○ **What is thyrotoxicosis, and what are its causes?**

A hypermetabolic state that occurs secondary to excess circulating thyroid hormone caused by thyroid hormone overdose, thyroid hyperfunction, or thyroid inflammation.

○ **What are the clinical features of myxedema coma?**

Hypothermia (75%), and unconsciousness.

○ **A patient who is on chronic steroids presents with weakness, depression, fatigue, and postural dizziness. What pathological process should be suspected? What is the treatment?**

Adrenal insufficiency. The treatment is to administer large "stress doses" of steroids and rule out any serious medical problems.

○ **Are diabetic patients on oral hypoglycemics, who mix their medication with alcohol, more likely to become hyper or hypoglycemic?**

Hypoglycemic.

○ **What key lab results are expected with SIADH?**

Low serum sodium levels and high urine sodium levels (i.e., >30).

○ **What electrolyte disorder is associated with hypercalcemia?**

Hypokalemia.

○ **What drug will most rapidly lower serum potassium levels?**

Calcium chloride IV (1–3 minutes). Remember that CaCl is very toxic to tissue and if extravasation of the IV occurs, there may be severe skin necrosis. Consider use of a central line when using CaCl. If any doubt about the peripheral IV exists, the nurse should consider using calcium gluconate instead, which requires metabolism by the liver in order to free up the calcium.

○ **What is a potential side effect of the use of kayexalate?**

Kayexalate exchanges sodium for K+. As a result, sodium overload and CHF may occur.

○ **An elderly patient presents with altered mental status, history of IDDM, and is hypoglycemic. Core temperature is 32°C. What endocrinologic condition is likely?**

Myxedema coma. Other clues to look for are history of thyroid surgery, hypothyroidism, and use of antithyroid medications.

○ **What are the signs and symptoms of myxedema coma?**

Lethargy, stupor, decreased level of consciousness, delayed deep tendon reflexes, progressive respiratory depression, weight gain, hypoglycemia, dry skin and hair, and hypothermia.

○ **You dipstick the diabetic client's urine and it tests positive for acetone. What does this indicate?**

The development of ketoacidosis resulting from the body's breakdown of fats. This occurs in DKA, patients with vomiting and/or lack of eating food, and other situations.

○ **What electrolyte can become depleted when a patient is on Lasix therapy?**

Potassium. Most patients who take Lasix chronically will need potassium supplements to maintain proper potassium levels.

○ **Interpret the following blood gases: pH 7.49, $PaCO_2$ 36, HCO_3 40, PaO_2 92.**

Metabolic alkalosis.

○ **Interpret the following blood gases: pH 7.30, $PaCO_2$ 40, HCO_3 20, PaO_2 95.**

Metabolic acidosis.

○ **What blood test can help determine if your client's intake of protein is adequate?**

Serum albumin.

○ **What electrolyte imbalance can cause digoxin toxicity?**

Hypokalemia.

○   **What electrolyte and fluid changes would you expect in a patient with syndrome of inappropriate antidiuretic hormone (SIADH)?**

Hypervolemia and dilutional hyponatremia due to an excess of antidiuretic hormone (ADH).

○   **Why should hypoglycemia be considered dangerous and treated immediately?**

It can lead to brain damage, coma, and even death.

○   **A medsurg nurse is taking care of a newly admitted diabetic patient. The 60-year-old lady complains of confusion, and says her left arm is very weak. In addition to considering a stroke, what test should be done immediately to rule out a reversible problem?**

Obtain a STAT accu-check or blood sugar level to rule out hypoglycemia.

○   **What precautions should you take if a patient's potassium level rises to a dangerous level?**

Place the patient on a cardiac monitor and prepare for the possibility of cardiac arrest.

○   **What does a positive Trousseau's sign indicate?**

Hypocalcemia. Trousseau's sign is when a blood pressure cuff is used to occlude the brachial artery by inflating to a pressure greater than the systolic blood pressure and held in place for 3 minutes. If carpal spasm (flexion at the wrist and metacarpophalangeal joints, with extension of the DIP and PIP finger joints) occurs, then the patient likely has hypocalcemia. It is less sensitive than the Chvostek's sign (twitching of facial muscles/lips when the facial nerve is tapped at the angle of the jaw).

○   **What is the appropriate needle size for an insulin injection?**

25 gauge and 5/8 inch (1.5 cm) long.

○   **What medication can be given via enema to lower an elevated potassium level?**

Sodium polystyrene sulfonate (kayexalate). The dose is 15–60 g every 4–6 hours as needed to treat hyperkalemia.

○   **What is the normal BUN value?**

10–20 mg/dl.

○   **What are the causes of a metabolic acidosis?**

Diabetic ketoacidosis, lactic acidosis, diarrhea, renal failure, toxic drug ingestion, extreme physical activity, and high doses of acetazolamide.

○   **What medication should be given to a patient who is hypoglycemic and unconscious?**

IV glucose (dextrose) if an IV line is available. If not, an IM injection of glucagons 1 mg will help reverse the hypoglycemia. Monitor for recurrence of hypoglycemia.

○   **What are the findings in a patient with diabetic ketoacidosis?**

Polyuria, polydipsia, anorexia, muscle cramps and vomiting, Kussmaul's respirations, stupor, and coma.

○ **A medsurg nurse admits a patient with Addison's disease. What is the *most common* cause of this chronic adrenocortical insuffiency?**

Autoimmune destruction of the adrenal cortex. Other causes include infection, hemorrhage, and metastatic disease.

○ **What syndrome causes primary Addison's disease?**

This results from low levels of glucocorticoids and mineralocorticoids.

○ **What is secondary Addison's disease?**

Secondary Addison's disease results from inadequate pituitary secretion of corticotrophin.

○ **Describe Cushing's syndrome.**

Cushing's syndrome is abnormally high function of the adrenal cortex caused by an overabundance of cortisol. Cortisol-dependent Cushing's is caused in 80% of cases by a pituitary adenoma. Cortisol-independent Cushing's syndrome is usually caused by a tumor in the adrenal cortex or islet cell tumor.

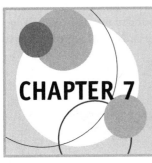

CHAPTER 7 Neurology Pearls

○ **A 35-year-old woman with a history of flu like symptoms (URI) 1 week ago, now presents with vertigo, nausea, and vomiting. No auditory impairment or focal deficits are noted. What is the most likely cause of her problem?**

Labyrinthitis or vestibular neuronitis.

○ **During a routine Romberg exam, a patient is asked to stand with his eyes open. He falls to the left. What do you suspect?**

Cerebellar dysfunction. An unsteady, broad-based gait suggests cerebellar problems. If the patient only falls with eyes closed, the problem is with sensation, usually as a result of abnormality in position sense, most commonly posterior column dysfunction.

○ **There are several types of migraine headaches. Describe the key signs and symptoms of classic, common, cluster, ophthalmoplegic, and hemiplegic migraine headache.**

Classic: Prodrome lasts up to 60 minutes. Most common symptom is visual disturbance, such as homonymous hemianopsia, scintillating scotoma, and photophobia. Lips, face, and hand tingling as well as aphasia and extremity weakness may occur. Nausea and vomiting may also occur.

Common: Most common. Slow evolving headache over hours to days. A positive family history as well as two of the following: nausea or vomiting, throbbing quality, photophobia, unilateral pain, and increase with menses. Distinguishing feature from "Classic" migraine is the lack of visual symptoms.

Cluster: Mostly males. Intense unilateral ocular or retroocular pain which lasts less than 2 hours and occurs several times a day for weeks or months. Symptoms include lacrimation, facial flushing, rhinorrhea, sweating, and conjunctival injection. Often awakes patient from sleep.

Ophthalmoplegic: Most commonly seen in young adults. Patient has an outwardly deviated, dilated eye, with ptosis. The 3rd > 6th > 4th nerves are typically involved.

Hemiplegic: Unilateral motor and sensory symptoms, mild hemiparesis to hemiplegia.

○ **Treatment of a cluster headache?**

Preventive treatment with beta blockers, calcium channel blockers, certain anticonvulsants; abortive treatments include trial of 100% O_2, ergotamine, triptan drugs, 4% lidocaine in the ipsilateral nostril, and/or a short course of steroids.

○ **A 29-year-old drunken male is admitted for observation after having his head pounded into the concrete by his wife. The patient had a brief episode of LOC, but was then ambulatory and alert. Now he appears drowsy and just threw up on you. What do you suspect?**

Epidural hematoma.

○ **A 25-year-old presents with a history of being knocked unconscious for 10 seconds while playing touch football 1 week ago. Since then he has felt malaise, intermittent vertigo, nausea, vomiting, blurred vision, and a headache. Neuro exam and CT are normal. What do you suspect?**

Postconcussion syndrome, including post-traumatic vertigo. Expect recovery to normal over 2–6 weeks. These patients should refrain from sports or any activity that may produce another concussion until cleared by a competent physician. Cumulative brain trauma has an exponentially worse outcome when repeated before healing.

○ **A 53-year-old female presents with unilateral right-sided sudden onset lancinating pain in the distribution of the second and third branches of the fifth cranial nerve. What syndrome does this describe?**

Trigeminal neuralgia. Treatment includes appropriate diagnosis and use of carbamazepine (Tegretol).

○ **A 28-year-old woman raised in Minnesota complains of weakness and tingling in the right arm and leg for 2 days. She reports an episode of right eye pain and blurred vision, which resolved over one mo that occurred 2 years ago. She also recalls a 2-week episode of intermittent blurred vision 1 year ago. What disease process could be present?**

Multiple sclerosis (MS). She could be experiencing optic neuritis, a symptom of MS.

○ **A 50-year-old female presents with acute vertigo, nausea, and vomiting. She reports similar episodes over the last 20 years, sometimes but not always associated with hearing change and/or hearing loss and tinnitus. She has permanent right > left sensorineural hearing loss. Diagnosis?**

Ménière's disease.

○ **What is the *most common* cause of a subarachnoid hemorrhage?**

Leakage or rupture of a brain aneurysm.

○ **A 42-year-old air traffic controller is admitted with dizziness. He has had attacks of vertigo whenever he scans the skies for landing airplanes. Symptoms last about a minute. Neuro exam is normal. What do you tell him about his disease?**

Nothing until a diagnosis is made, even though you suspect benign positional vertigo as the symptoms are associated with head movement.

○ **A patient is admitted with acute meningitis; when should antibiotics be initiated?**

Immediately. Do not wait. Bring this patient to the physician's attention immediately if you suspect this diagnosis.

○ **What is the *most common* presenting symptom of MS?**

Optic neuritis (about 25%).

○ **What rhythm disturbance would make phenytoin relatively contraindicated?**

Second- or third-degree heart block. If the patient is in status epilepticus, you may have no choice.

○ **What three bacterial illness present with peripheral neurologic findings?**

Botulism, tetanus, and diphtheria.

○ **What is the most likely cause of unilateral transient loss of vision in a patient's eye (amaurosis fugax)?**

Carotid artery disease. This is usually the result of platelet emboli from plaques in the arterial system.

○ **Differentiate between decerebrate and decorticate posturing.**

Decerebrate: Elbows and legs are extended which is indicative of a midbrain lesion.
Decorticate: Elbows are flexed, legs are extended. This suggests a lesion in the thalamic region.

○ **A 32-year-old female complains of periods of weakness, especially when she chews her food. She presents with ptosis, diplopia, and dysarthria. Her muscles weaken with repetitive exercise. What neurological condition does this describe?**

Myasthenia gravis. A patient with myasthenia gravis produces autoimmune antibodies against her own acetylcholine receptors in the neuromuscular junction.

○ **A resting tremor is most likely related to what disease?**

Parkinson's disease. The tremors of Parkinson's disease are generally asymmetrical and have the characteristic "pill rolling" appearance.

○ **Describe the key features of Ménière's disease, also known as endolymphatic hydrops.**

Vertigo, hearing loss, and tinnitus are the hallmarks of Ménière's disease. Ménière's disease typically presents with the rapid onset of vertigo and nausea/vomiting that lasts from hours to 1 day. Nystagmus may be spontaneous during the critical stage. Tinnitus may be present and is louder during the attacks. Sensorineural hearing loss may occur. There may also be an aura with a sensation of fullness in the ear during an attack. Symptoms are unilateral in over 90% of patients, and recurring attacks are typical.

○ **What is the treatment for Wernicke's encephalopathy?**

Thiamine given intravenously.

○ **Why would you be concerned if a quadriplegic suddenly develops a severe headache?**

It is a symptom of autonomic dysreflexia. Bladder distension is one of the most common causes.

○ **What does the term "stroke in evolution" mean?**

A stroke in which neurologic changes continue to occur for 24–48 hours after the initial incident.

○ **A client with right-sided hemiplegia following a stroke is most likely to have difficulty seeing objects to which side of the body?**

The right side.

○ **Difficulty in speaking and understanding speech is often associated with a stroke to which hemisphere of the brain?**

Left.

○ **A common adverse effect of aminoglycoside therapy is what type of neurological damage?**

Damage to the 8th cranial nerve.

○ **What is believed to be the cause of pain in migraine headaches?**

Dilation of the cranial arteries.

○ **What purpose would the drug baclofen (Lioresal) serve when administered to a patient with multiple sclerosis?**

It is a muscle relaxant used to help relieve muscle spasms common with MS.

○ **What is the classic gait exhibited by a patient with Parkinson's disease?**

A shuffling, propulsive gait.

○ **What are important nursing actions if a patient is having a grand mal seizure?**

Protect the head, protect him/her from injury, move furniture away from flailing arms and legs, maintain a patent airway, and start an IV line.

○ **What behavior would you expect from a patient following a seizure?**

The patient is usually disoriented and tired (postictal), sleeping for a long period of time and incontinent.

○ **A widening pulse pressure is an indication of what neurologic disorder?**

Increased intercranial pressure (ICP).

○ **What is the earliest sign of increased intracranial pressure (ICP)?**

An altered level of consciousness (increased ICP).

○ **What is the calculation for cerebral perfusion pressure (CPP)?**

Cerebral perfusion pressure is the pressure at which the brain cells are perfused. CPP = MAP − ICP (mean arterial pressure minus ICP) CPP is normally 60 mm Hg.

○ **What respiratory pattern is indicative of increased intercranial pressure?**

Slow, irregular respirations.

○ **T/F: For patients with increased intracranial pressure due to trauma or tumor, it is recommended that all patients be hyperventilated.**

False; the old school thought was to hyperventilate the patient, which decreased the blood volume and this lowered the ICP. This has since been proven to be associated with a worse outcome except in rare circumstances where a patient suddenly produces a mass-effect with intracranial bleeding and midline shift, at risk for herniation of the brainstem. Hyperventilation actually may later increase the blood flow when the vasoconstriction reverses.

○ **What is the purpose of administering ergotamine (Gynergen) to a patient with a migraine?**

Stop the migraine attack by causing vasoconstriction of the dilated vessels.

○   **Describe the three phases of seizures.**

Prodromal phase: occurs before the seizure and produces auras (sensory signals that warn of an approaching seizure) such as sudden slash of light, or smell sensation, or slight behavior changes. The second phase is the ictal phase which is the seizure itself. The third phase is the postictal phase, after the seizure has ended and may last for minutes or hours.

○   **T/F: A 24-year-old female begins seizing for the 4th time, and initial treatment is to insert a tongue blade or bite block to prevent her from biting her tongue?**

False. Although the airway should be maintained, this rarely is a problem. Forcing a tongue blade or other object into the patient's mouth may break her teeth.

○   **What side effect will likely manifest if a patient who is on phenytoin (Dilantin) suddenly stops taking the drug?**

Status epilepticus.

○   **What type of seizure would be described as a sudden stiffening of the muscles followed by rhythmic, violent muscle contractions.**

Tonic-clonic or grand mal seizure.

○   **What is the term for a sensory premonition prior to a seizure?**

An aura.

○   **What is the primary cause of new onset seizures in adults over the age of 20?**

Trauma.

○   **What side of the brain has a stroke most likely affected if a patient has expressive aphasia?**

The left side. A left-hemispheric stroke causes expressive aphasia, global or receptive aphasia (most people have the left side dominant for speech), right-sided hemiparesis, and slow, cautious behavior.

○   **What position is contraindicated for a patient with a herniated disc and why?**

Prone, because hyperextension places the most strain on the spine.

○   **What are some common symptoms of a herniated lumbar disc?**

Back pain relieved by rest, a change in deep tendon reflexes, and activities that increase spinal fluid pressure such as sneezing, coughing, and bending cause increased pain.

○   **What is the medical treatment for Ménière's disease?**

Many treatments are used including diuretics, antihistamines, anticholinergics, and a low sodium diet.

○   **Prior to an attack of Ménière's disease, what sensation does the patient often complain of?**

A feeling of fullness from the developing congestion.

○   **In what part of the spine do herniated intervertebral discs most commonly occur?**

Lumbar and lumbosacral region.

○   **What is tardive dyskinesia?**

Involuntary, repetitive movements of the tongue, lips, extremities, and trunk.

○   **What is the most serious complication in a patient who has had an acute stroke?**

Increasing ICP and subsequent brain damage.

○   **What does the term "oriented times 3" indicate?**

The patient is alert and oriented to person, place, and time.

○   **What is Bell's palsy?**

Unilateral facial weakness or paralysis that is caused by disturbance of the seventh cranial nerve.

○   **What is the major complication of Bell's palsy?**

Corneal inflammation (keratitis). All patients should get a careful slit lamp and fluorescein stain eye exam performed to rule out viral dendrites, which untreated can severely damage the eyes.

○   **What does the term "ataxia" refer to?**

An impaired ability to coordinate movement.

○   **Differentiate between Korsakoff's psychosis and Wernicke's encephalopathy.**

Korsakoff's psychosis: Inability to process new information (i.e., to form new memories). This is a reversible condition resulting from brain damage induced by a thiamine deficiency which is generally secondary to chronic alcoholism.

Wernicke's encephalopathy: This disease is also due to an alcoholic-induced thiamine deficiency. It is an irreversible disease in which the brain tissues break down, become inflamed and bleed. Patients have decreased muscle coordination, ophthalmoplegia, and confusion.

○   **Differentiate between dementia and delirium.**

Dementia: Irreversible impaired functioning secondary to changes/deficits in memory, spatial concepts, personality, cognition, language, motor and sensory skills, judgment, or behavior. There is no change in consciousness.

Delirium: A reversible organic mental syndrome reflecting deficits in attention, organized thinking, orientation, speech, memory and perception. Patients are frequently confused, anxious, excited and have hallucinations. A change in consciousness can be observed.

○   **T/F: Alzheimer's disease is a memory-related disease that is reversible with medications.**

False. Alzheimer's disease is a progressive degenerative disorder of the brain that is irreversible. The exact cause is unknown; initial stages include recent memory loss and impaired judgment, inability to learn and retain new information, and difficulty finding words; later stages include decreased abililty to care for self, wandering, agitation and hostility, and possibly eventually inability to walk, incontinence, and no intelligible speech. Medications may help improve memory in early stages, but there is no cure. It is typically diagnosed when other dementia-producing conditions have been ruled out.

○   **What is the *most common* cause of drug-induced hallucinations in the geriatric population?**

Propranolol.

○ **An acute confusional state is also known as?**

Delirium. Diagnostic features include reduced level of consciousness, disorganized sleep-wake cycles, disturbances in attention, global cognitive impairment and decreased or increased psychomotor activity.

○ **What are the two major causes of dementia?**

Alzheimer's disease and multi-infarction. Demented patients may have decreased memory, cognition, language ability, judgment, and sensory and motor function. There is no change is consciousness, although personality changes do exist.

○ **A 20-year-old male is admitted with ingestion of unknown drugs and acute psychosis. Name some over-the-counter and "street" drugs that may produce delirium or acute psychosis.**

Salicylates, antihistamines, anticholinergics, alcohols, phencyclidine, LSD, mescaline, cocaine, and amphetamines.

○ **What are the signs and symptoms suggestive of an organic source of psychosis.**

Acute onset, disorientation, visual or tactile hallucinations, age less than 10 or older than 60, and evidence suggesting overdose or acute ingestion, such as abnormal vital signs, pupil size, and reactivity (or nystagmus).

○ **What is a dystonic reaction?**

It is a common side effect of neuroleptic drugs (approximately 2%). Extraparamidal effects including spasm of the tongue, face, neck, and back are seen. Severe laryngospasm and extraocular muscle spasm may also occur.

○ **How do you treat a dystonic reaction?**

Diphenhydramine (Benadryl), 25–50 mg IM or IV or benztropine (Cogentin), 1–2 mg IV or PO. Remember that dystonias can recur acutely, so patients should take the above medicines for several days.

○ **What pathology should be presumed when there is a sudden loss of bladder control, onset of lumbosacral pain, and associated bilateral leg pain?**

Midline herniation of a thoracolumbar disk. With these symptoms comes the threat of paraparesis. Severe compression can result in cauda equine syndrome.

○ **What are some common symptoms of a herniated lumbar disc?**

Back pain relieved by rest, a change in deep tendon reflexes and activities that increase spinal fluid pressure such as sneezing, coughing, and bending cause increased pain.

○ **What common neuroleptic drug can sometimes induce a dystonic reaction?**

Compazine.

○ **What cranial nerve controls movement of the tongue?**

Cranial nerve XII-Hypoglossal.

○ **A trauma patient with a suspected head injury complains of pain. What narcotic should be given to this patient?**

None. Until a head injury is ruled out, narcotics are avoided because of the effects on level consciousness, respiratory rate, and blood pressure.

○   **What is the length of time it can take for Battle sign to become evident after a basilar skull fracture?**

12–24 hours.

○   **At what level of spinal injury will a patient be unable to breathe on his own?**

C-2. The diaphragm is innervated by C-3, C-4, C-5. "C-3, 4, 5 keep your diaphragm alive" is one way to memorize this.

○   **At what level of spinal injury will a patient be considered a paraplegic?**

T-1–L-2.

○   **What simple nursing interventions can help decrease ICP?**

Head of bed elevated 15–30 degrees, decreasing stimuli and pain, avoiding pressure on the eyes, avoiding neck flexion, avoiding straining such as reaching, and avoid the Valsalva's maneuver.

○   **The patient with personality changes is found to have a brain tumor. What area of the brain is most likely to be found in?**

Frontal lobe.

○   **What part of the brain is responsible for respiratory and cardiac function?**

Medulla.

○   **When administering large amount of diazepam (Valium), what life-threatening side effect should the nurse be aware of?**

Respiratory depression. Pulse oximetry should be used in any patient with possible respiratory compromise.

○   **A patient is admitted who complains of nausea, vomiting, photosensitivity, and difficulty in speaking. She says this is "The worst headache of my life." There is no history of migraines. What priority should this patient receive?**

Immediate. Suspect a ruptured cerebral aneurysm until proven otherwise. A CT brain scan should be performed in most circumstances, and if this is normal, should be followed by a lumbar puncture to evaluate the CSF fluid for blood.

○   **What is usually the earliest indicator of a change in neurologic status?**

A change in level of consciousness.

○   **Contraindications to lumber puncture:**

Increased intracranial pressure, mass in the brain with shift, recent thrombolytic therapy, infection at the puncture site, or significant coagulopathy.

○   **The inability to make sounds that are understandable is called:**

Expressive aphasia.

○ **Priority nursing diagnosis for the patient with increased intracranial pressure?**

Altered cerebral tissue perfusion.

○ **A nursing diagnosis for the client with Alzheimer's?**

Potential for injury related to confusion.

○ **A patient with Myasthenia gravis is admitted to the floor with suspected anticholinesterase toxicity. What drug is given to reverse effects?**

Atropine.

○ **Symptoms of postconcussion syndrome:**

Headache, dizziness, irritability, insomnia, nausea, vomiting, and difficulty in concentrating.

○ **What is normal intracranial pressure reading?**

Less than 10 mm Hg.

○ **What physical manifestations are present with increased ICP?**

Cheyne-Stokes respiration, widened pulse pressure, hyperthermia, and decreased level of consciousness.

○ **What reflex can help evaluate brain stem function in an unconscious patient?**

Oculocephalic reflex (doll's eyes).

○ **What is the definition of CVA?**

Cerebrovascular accident, which is a disruption in cerebral circulation, causing permanent neurologic deficits. There are several types. An occlusive stroke may occur from an embolism, vasospasm, or atherosclerotic placque that ruptures. A thrombotic ischemic stroke occurs when there is partial to complete occlusion, and may be preceded by a TIA (transient ischemic attack). A hemorrhagic stroke may occur due to ruptures AVM (ateriovenous malformation), aneurysm, trauma, arterial rupture, or bleeding disorder. Symptoms vary with the distribution of the cerebral artery affected.

○ **What are the cardinal signs and symptoms of meningitis?**

Infection symptoms and increased ICP (intracranial pressure), including fever, chills, malaise, headache, nausea, vomiting, irritability, change in level of consciousness, and seizures.

○ **What is Brudzinski sign?**

Physical exam finding in a patient with meningitis; when the neck if flexed forward, then leg adduction and flexion occur.

○ **What is Kernig's sign?**

Physical exam finding in a patient with meningitis; when the thigh is flexed up to the abdomen, there is resistance to extension of the lower leg, due to meningeal irritation.

○   **What is MS (multiple sclerosis)?**

MS is a progressive neurologic disease that is not infectious, and is caused by destruction, injury, or malformation of the myelin sheaths that cover nerves; these areas of demyelination are called plaques and are most common on the white matter of the brain and spinal cord; symptoms of MS may be transient, variable, and bizarre. The first symptoms are usually sensory and visual problems. Fatigue is usually the most debilitating symptom. Diagnosis is by MRI and other techniques. There is no cure, although medical treatment does help symptoms, including steroids, glatiramer acetate, and others.

○   **A patient with a C-6 spinal cord injury is admitted to the medsurg floor. The patient develops bradycardia, hypertension, and sweating. What is the possible diagnosis, and what should the nurse do at this time?**

Autonomic dysreflexia is a complication of complete spinal cord injury; injuries above T6 are at greatest risk; this is a clinical emergency caused by stimulation of the autonomic reflexes below the level of the lesion; severe hypertension, bradycardia, pale skin with pilomotor spasm (goose bumps/hair erection), blotchy skin, diaphoresis, headache, and vasodilation above the lesion level may be seen; it may be precipitated by a full bladder or rectum, painful stimuli, skin stimulation, and visceral contractions (bladder spasms, pregnancy). Treatment includes stopping or removing the sensory stimulus and medication control of the high blood pressure.

○   **What should a medsurg nurse do to prevent increases in ICP in a patient admitted with a closed head injury?**

Elevate the head of the bed 15–40 degrees, avoid suctioning the patient or other stimulation, maintaining a quiet and dimly lit room, and use of sedation if indicated to prevent overstimulation of patient.

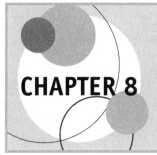

CHAPTER 8

Infectious Disease/ Rheumatology/ Immunology Pearls

○ **Describe the pathophysiologic features of HIV.**

HIV (human immunodeficiency virus) is a virus that selectively infects cells with a CD4+ surface marker, usually T4 helper cells. HIV is a single-stranded RNA retrovirus. HIV has been found in saliva, urine, cerebrospinal fluid, tears, alveolar fluid, synovial fluid, breast milk, and amniotic fluid. It destroys T4 lymphocytes, and increases the patient's susceptibility to opportunistic infections and cancers.

○ **How quickly do patients infected with HIV become symptomatic?**

5–10% develop symptoms within 3 years of seroconversion. Predictive characteristics include low T4 count, and hematocrit less than 40. Mean incubation time is about 8 years for adults and 2 years for children less than 5.

○ **Name the *most common* causes of fever in HIV infected patients:**

HIV-related fever, Mycobacterium avium-intracellulare, CMV, non-Hodgkin's and Hodgkin's lymphoma.

○ **An HIV positive patient presents with a history of weight loss, diarrhea, fever, anorexia, and malaise and is also dyspneic. Lab studies reveal abnormal LFTs and anemia. Diagnosis?**

Mycobacterium avium-intracellulare. Lab confirmation is made by acid-fast stain of body fluids or by blood culture.

○ **What is the *most common* cause of retinitis in AIDS patients?**

CMV (cytomegalovirus). GI involvement is also common. Findings include photophobia, redness, scotoma, pain, or change in visual acuity. On exam, findings include fluffy white retinal lesions.

○ **What is the second *most common* complication of AIDS?**

Kaposi's sarcoma. Pneumocystis carinii pneumonia (PCP) is the *most common.*

○ **What is the *most common* cause of focal encephalitis in AIDS patients?**

Toxoplasmosis. Symptoms include focal neurologic deficits, headache, fever, altered mental status, and seizures. Ring enhancing-lesions are seen on CT.

○ **The differential diagnosis of ring-enhancing lesions seen on CT scan of the brain in AIDS patients is:**

Lymphoma, cerebral tuberculosis, fungal infection, CMV, Kaposi's sarcoma, toxoplasmosis, and hemorrhage.

○ **What are the signs and symptoms of CNS cryptococcal infection in an AIDS patient?**

Headache, depression, lightheadedness, seizures, and cranial nerve palsies. Diagnosis is made by India ink prep, fungal culture, or by cryptococcal antigen in the CSF.

○ **What is the *most common* opportunistic infection in AIDS patients?**

PCP. Symptoms may include nonproductive cough and dyspnea. Chest x-ray may show diffuse interstitial infiltrates or be negative. Gallium scanning is more sensitive but results in false positives. Initial treatment includes TMP-SMX. Pentamidine is an alternative.

○ **A patient is infected with Treponema pallidum, what is the treatment?**

Syphilis is treated with benzathine penicillin G, 2.4 million units IM or tetracycline 500 mg qid po for 15 days, or erythromycin 500 mg qid po for 15 days.

○ **What is the incubation period in tetanus?**

Hours to over 1 month. The shorter the incubation, the more severe the disease. Most patients in the United States who get the disease are over 50.

○ **What is the *most common* presentation of tetanus?**

"Generalized tetanus" with pain and stiffness in the trunk and jaw muscles. Trismus develops and results in risus sardonicus (sardonic smile).

○ **What cranial nerve is most commonly involved in cephalic tetanus?**

Cephalic tetanus usually occurs after injuries to the head and typically involves the 7th cranial nerve.

○ **Explain the pathophysiology of rabies:**

Infection occurs within the myocytes for the first 48–96 hours. It then spreads across the motor endplate, ascends and replicates along peripheral nervous axoplasm into the dorsal root ganglia, the spinal cord, and CNS. From the gray matter, the virus spreads by peripheral nerves to tissues and organ systems.

○ **What are the signs and symptoms of rabies?**

Initial: fever, headache, malaise, anorexia, sore throat, nausea, cough, and pain or paresthesias at the bite site.

CNS stage: agitation, restlessness, altered mental status, painful bulbar and peripheral muscular spasms, bulbar or focal motor paresis, and opisthotonos. Similar to Landry-Guillain-Barré syndrome, 20% develop ascending, symmetric flaccid and areflexic paralysis. Hypersensitivity to water and sensory stimuli (light, touch, and noise) may occur.

Progressive stage: lucid and confused intervals with hyperpyrexia, lacrimation, salivation, and mydriasis may occur along with brainstem dysfunction, hyperreflexia and extensor plantar response.

Final stage: coma, convulsions, and apnea, followed by death at days 4–7 in the untreated patient.

○ **How is rabies treated?**

RIG 20 IU/kg, half at wound site and half in the DELTOID muscle. HDCV 1-ml doses IM on days 0,3,7,14, and 28 also in the DELTOID muscle on the opposite side of the body, away from the RIG.

○   **What is the second *most common* tick borne disease?**

Rocky Mountain spotted fever (RMSF).

Causative agent—Rickettsia rickettsii.

Vector—Female Ixodi ticks, *Dermacentor andersonii* (wood tick), and *D. variabilis* (American dog tick).

○   **A patient is admitted to the medsurg floor presenting with fever up to 40°C followed by a rash which is erythematous, macular, and blanching. The rash progresses to deep red, dusky, papular and becomes petechial. The patient also complains of a headache, vomiting, myalgias, and cough. Where did the rash begin?**

RMSF rash typically begins on the flexor surfaces of the ankles and wrists and spreads centripetally and centrifugally.

○   **What is the most deadly form of malaria?**

Plasmodium falciparum.

○   **What is the vector for malaria?**

The female anopheline mosquito.

○   **What lab findings would you expect in a patient with malaria?**

Normochromic normocytic anemia, normal or depressed leukocyte count, thrombocytopenia, an elevated sed rate, abnormal kidney and LFTs, hyponatremia, hypoglycemia, and false-positive VDRL.

○   **What is the drug of choice for treating *P. vivax, P. ovale,* and *P. malariae*?**

Chloroquine.

○   **What is the *most common* intestinal parasite in the United States?**

Giardia. Cysts are obtained from contaminated water or passed by hand-to-mouth transmission. Symptoms include explosive foul smelling diarrhea, abdominal distension, fever, fatigue, and weight loss. Cysts reside in the duodenum and upper jejunum. Treatment is quinacrine.

○   **What two diseases do the deer tick, *Ixodes dammini,* transmit?**

Lyme disease and babesiosis.

○   **What is the most frequently transmitted tick-borne disease?**

Lyme disease.
Causative agent: spirochete, *Borrelia burgdorferi.*
Vector: *Ixodes dammini* (deer tick) also *I. pacificus, Amblyomma americanum,* and *Dermacentor variabilis.*

○   **When are patients most likely to acquire Lyme disease?**

Late spring and late summer, peaks in July.

○   **How is Lyme disease diagnosed?**

Immunofluorescent and immunoabsorbent assays diagnose the antibodies to the spirochete.

Treatment includes doxycycline or tetracycline, amoxicillin, IV penicillin V in pregnant patients, or erythromycin.

○ **What is a paronychia?**

An infection of the lateral nail fold. Usually from S. aureus or Streptococcus. Treat with I&D followed by warm soaks.

○ **What type of paralysis does tick paralysis cause?**

Ascending paralysis. The venom, which causes paralysis, is probably a neurotoxin which causes a conduction block at the peripheral motor nerve branches. This prevents acetylcholine release at the neuromuscular junction. Forty three species of ticks are implicated as causative agents.

○ **A patient is admitted with sudden onset of fever, lethargy, headache, myalgias, anorexia, nausea and vomiting. They describe the headache as retro-orbital and are extremely photophobic. They have been on a camping trip in Wyoming. What tick-borne disease might cause these symptoms?**

Colorado tick fever is caused by a virus of the genus orbivirus of the family Reoviridae. The vector is the tick *D. andersoni*. The disease is self-limited and treatment is supportive.

○ **A high level of hepatitis B serum marker (HBsAg) 3 months after the onset of acute hepatitis B infection suggests what?**

The development of chronic hepatitis or a carrier state.

○ **What groups of people are at high risk for hepatitis B exposure?**

IV drug users, multiple sex partners, health care workers exposed to blood, and homosexuals.

○ **Hairy leukoplakia is characteristic of what two viruses?**

HIV and Epstein-Barr virus. Hairy leukoplakia is usually found on the lateral aspect of the tongue.

○ **What is the *most common* oral manifestation of AIDS?**

Oropharyngeal thrush. Other AIDS-related oropharyngeal diseases include Kaposi's sarcoma, hairy leukoplakia, and non-Hodgkin's lymphoma.

○ **What is the *most common* cause of bacterial diarrhea?**

E. coli (enteroinvasive, enteropathogenic, enterotoxigenic).

○ **Which is the *most common* form of acute diarrhea?**

Viral diarrhea. It is generally self-limited, lasting only 1–3 days.

○ **What is the most probable cause of diarrhea that develops within 12 hours of a meal?**

An ingested preformed toxin.

○ **When does traveler's diarrhea typically occur?**

3–7 days after arrival in a foreign land.

○ **You stick yourself with a needle from a chronic hepatitis B carrier. You've been vaccinated, but have never had your antibody status checked. What is the appropriate postexposure prophylaxis?**

Measure your anti-HB's titer. If it is adequate (>10 mIU), treatment is not required. If it is inadequate, you'll need a vaccine booster and a single dose of HBIG as soon as possible. Nurses and other hospital employees should undergo appropriate support and counseling, including consideration of HIV risks, source patient testing, and possibly starting a 1-month PEP (postexposure prophylaxis) medicine dosage aimed at decreasing chances of an HIV infection (if started within 2–3 hours can decrease incidence of an HIV/AIDS infection by 67%). Further followup, medication, and blood testing should be arranged.

○ **Name the *most common* causes of fever in HIV-infected patients.**

HIV related fever, including Mycobacterium avium intracellulare, CMV, and non-Hodgkin's and Hodgkin's lymphoma.

○ **What is the *most common* cause of focal encephalitis in AIDS patients?**

Toxoplasmosis. Symptoms include focal neurologic deficits, headache, fever, altered mental status, and seizures. Ring enhancing lesions are evident on CT.

○ **What is the *most common* opportunistic infection in AIDS patients?**

PCP. Symptoms may include a nonproductive cough and dyspnea. A chest x-ray may reveal diffused interstitial infiltrates or it may be negative.

○ **What is the *most common* gastrointestinal complaint in AIDS patients?**

Diarrhea. Hepatomegaly and hepatitis are also typical. Cryptosporidium and isospora are common causes of prolonged watery diarrhea.

○ **What is the risk of contracting HIV infection after an occupational exposure?**

0.32% for needle sticks and 0.08% for mucous membrane exposure to high risk body fluids. Eighty percent of the occupational exposure-related infections are from needle sticks.

○ **What is the *most common* site of herpes simplex I virus infection?**

The lower lip. First, the lip itches and burns, then the small vesicle with the red base appears. These lesions are painful and can frequently recur since the virus remains in the sensory ganglia. Stress, sun, and illness generally trigger recurrences.

○ **A patient presents with fever, acute polyarthritis, and migratory arthritis a few weeks after a bout of Streptococcal pharyngitis. What disease should be suspected?**

Acute rheumatic fever. Although the early symptoms may be nonspecific, a physical exam eventually reveals signs of arthritis (60–75%), carditis (30%), choreiform movements (10%), erythema marginatum, or subcutaneous nodules.

○ **What medical treatment should be started after the diagnosis of acute rheumatic fever has been made?**

Penicillin or erythromycin should be given even if cultures for Group A Streptococcus are negative. High dose aspirin therapy is used at an initial dose of 75–100 mg/kg/day. Carditis or congestive heart failure is treated with prednisone, 1–2 mg/kg/day.

○ **How does the pain associated with epididymitis differ from that produced by prostatitis?**

Epididymitis: The pain begins in the scrotum or groin and radiates along the spermatic cord. It intensifies rapidly, is associated with dysuria, and is relieved with scrotal elevation (Prehn's sign).

Prostatitis: Patients will have frequency, dysuria, urgency, bladder outlet obstruction, and retention. They may have low back pain and perineal pain associated with fever, chills, arthralgias, and myalgias.

○ **A 19-year old male has been admitted for treatment of his gunshot wound. He complains of intense itching of the penis and the web spaces of his hands. What do you suspect?**

Scabies frequently attacks the web spaces of the hands and feet. Small vesicles and papules may be present.

○ **What infection carries the highest risk of transmission by blood transfusion?**

Hepatitis C.

○ ***Candida albicans* infections of the skin are most commonly located where?**

In the intertriginous areas (i.e., in the folds of the skin, axilla, groin, under the breasts, etc.) *Candida albicans* appears as a beefy red rash with satellite lesions.

○ **A mother brings her 18-year old boy to you a week after a physician prescribed ampicillin for his pharyngitis. Mom says he developed a rash over his torso, arms, legs, and even the palms of his hands. On examination, the patient has a erythematous, maculopapular rash in the places described. What might the child have other than pharyngitis?**

Infectious mononucleosis. In almost 95% of patients with Epstein-Barr viruses that are treated with ampicillin, a rash will develop. The rash and subsequent desquamation will last about a week.

○ **Where does a perirectal abscess originate?**

Anal crypts and burrows through the ischiorectal space. They may be perianal, perirectal, supralevator, or ischiorectal. Perianal abscesses, which involve the supralevator muscle, ischiorectal space, or rectum, require operative drainage.

○ **A 72-year old female presents complaining of a painful red rash with crops of blisters on erythematous bases in a band-like distribution on the right side of her lower back spreading down and out toward her hip. What do you suspect?**

Shingles or herpes zoster disease. This is due to a reactivation of the dormant varicella virus in the sensory root ganglia of a patient with a history of chickenpox. The rash is in the distribution of the dermatome, in this case L5. It is most common in the elderly population or in patients who are immunocompromised. Treatment is with acyclovir and oral analgesics. This will help decrease the postherpetic neuralgia that is frequently associated with the disease. The actual rash open sores contain chickenpox virus, and are thus contagious and should avoid pregnant women and children who may be immunocompromised or not yet undergone chickenpox immunization.

○ **Where is the *most common* site of eruption of herpes zoster?**

The thorax. Unlike chickenpox, shingles can recur.

○ **Tinea capitis is most commonly seen in what age group?**

Children aged 4–14. This is a fungal infection of the scalp that begins as a papule around one hair shaft and then spreads to other follicles. The infection can cause the hair to break off, leaving little black dot stumps and patches of alopecia. Trichophyton tonsurans is responsible for 90% of the cases. Wood's lamp examination will fluoresce only Microsporum infections, which are responsible for the remaining 10%. This is also called "ringworm of the scalp".

○ **What bacteria is the *most common* cause of UTIs in uncatheterized elderly patients?**

E. coli.

○ **What is the *most common* source of sepsis in the elderly?**

Respiratory > urinary > intra-abdominal.

○ **An 18-year old was just bitten by the neighbor's dog. She is frantic because she fears she will now develop rabies. What could you tell her to calm her fears?**

The incidence of rabies in the United States is 0–3 cases a year. The likelihood of infection is low. However, if the dog has not been vaccinated or appears ill, it should be quarantined for 10 days and observed.

○ **A patient presents with headache, fever, malaise, and tender regional lymphadenopathy about a week after a cat bite. A tender papule develops at the site. What diagnosis should be suspected by the nurse?**

Cat-scratch disease. This condition usually develops 3 days to 6 weeks following a cat bite or scratch. The papule typically blisters and heals with eschar formation. A transient macular or vesicular rash may also develop.

○ **What animals are the most prevalent vectors of rabies in the world? In the United States?**

Worldwide, the dog is the most common carrier of rabies.
In the United States, the skunk has become the most common carrier of disease. Bats, raccoons, cows, dogs, foxes, and cats (in descending order) are also sources. Most rabies victims who have died from bat rabies have no recollection of being bitten, but most remember being in or sleeping in a home with at least one bat flying around in the home. All household members should receive rabies prophylaxis until the animal can be caught and sent for analysis.

○ **How is hepatitis A transmitted?**

By the oral fecal route . . . i.e. poor hand-washing technique. No carrier state exists.

○ **Describe the symptoms and signs of varicella (chickenpox).**

The onset of varicella rash is 1–2 days after prodromal symptoms of slight malaise, anorexia, and fever. The rash begins on the trunk and scalp, appearing as faint macules which later become vesicles. Note that smallpox starts on the 'small parts' of the body (i.e., hands, feet) and spreads to the trunk.

○ **Who should receive prophylaxis after exposure to *Neisseria meningitidis*?**

People living with the patient or having close intimate contact. This includes medsurg nurses and other close contacts.

○ **When are clients with active TB considered to be noncontagious?**

After producing three consecutive sputum specimens that are free of M. tuberculosis.

○ **Following a diagnosis of active TB, the patient asks when he can return to work. How should you respond?**

As long as the patient is compliant with his medication, he will probably produce three negative sputum specimens within 2–3 weeks, at which time he may return to work.

○ **A nurse's aide refuses to go into an HIV positive client's room because she is afraid of contracting AIDS. How should you respond?**

Teach the aide how the HIV is transmitted and the concept of universal precautions.

○ **A patient with a positive TB skin test asks what that means. How should you respond?**

A positive skin test means that the patient has been exposed to tuberculosis. It does not mean the patient has the active disease. A chest x-ray and further examination will be needed to determine active TB.

○ **A client is taking isoniazid (INH) for active TB. You ask if he has had any right upper quadrant pain. Why?**

INH can cause liver dysfunction in some cases.

○ **A homeless client complains of night sweats, fever, cough, hemoptysis, pleuritic chest pain, and had a positive PPD skin test. What conclusions can you draw from this data?**

That the patient had been exposed to *M. tuberculosis*. Diagnosis of active TB is confirmed by chest x-ray and sputum samples.

○ **What is the mode of transmission for the tubercle bacillus?**

Inhalation of tubercle-laden droplets.

○ **What type of lab study is used to determine if the tubercle bacilli is present in sputum?**

Acid-fast staining.

○ **What is the general course of treatment for someone who has a positive Mantoux test, but does not have active TB?**

Oral isoniazid therapy for approximately 9 months.

○ **Why are clients often prescribed at least two drugs for the treatment of tuberculosis?**

It helps in reducing the development of resistant strains of the disease.

○ **What groups of people are at a high risk of developing tuberculosis today?**

The elderly, homeless, immunosuppressed/immunocompromised, foreign born from underdeveloped countries, and substance abusers.

○ **What types of patients are at increased risk for septic shock due to infection?**

The very young and the elderly, and the immunosuppressed.

○ **What common invasive device is a frequent cause of sepsis in the elderly?**

The Foley catheter.

○ **What is the mode of transmission for hepatitis B?**

Contact with blood or body fluids contaminated with the hepatitis B virus.

○ **What groups of people are at high risk for hepatitis B exposure?**

IV drug users, multiple sex partners, health care workers exposed to blood, and homosexuals.

○ **What is the purpose of prescribing probenecid (Benemid) along with penicillin?**

It inhibits the excretion of penicillin, thus higher serum levels of penicillin can be maintained for longer periods of time.

○ **Why should you be concerned when a HIV positive patient develops a herpes simplex infection?**

Herpes simplex is one of the AIDS defining illnesses. Its presence could indicate that the patient has converted to AIDS.

○ **What constitutes a positive tuberculin test?**

10 mm or more of induration at the injection site.

○ **A high level of hepatitis B serum marker (HBsAg) 3 months after the onset of acute hepatitis B infection suggests what?**

The development of chronic hepatitis or a carrier state.

○ **Why should a patient in the acute stage of infectious mononucleosis limit his physical exertion activities?**

To minimize the possibility of rupturing an enlarged spleen.

○ **Which protection items should be removed first when leaving an isolation room?**

Gloves and gown should be removed before the mask, because the mask carries fewer pathogens, and will provide continued protection as the gown and gloves are removed.

○ **What are some of the early physical signs of AIDS?**

Fever, pallor, anorexia, fatigue, night sweats, and large lymph nodes.

○ **What are the early signs and symptoms of tuberculosis?**

Low-grade fever, weight loss, night sweats, fatigue, cough, and anorexia.

○ **What is the *most common* symptom of hepatitis A?**

Anorexia.

○ **What is the primary reason for treating Streptococcal pharyngitis with antibiotics?**

To protect the heart valves and prevent rheumatic fever.

○ **What is the treatment of choice for a patient in anaphylactic shock?**

Epinephrine 0.3–0.5 mg IV of 1:10,000 solution. If no IV access, then inject into the venous plexus at base of the tongue.

○ **What is the *most common* cause of anaphylactoid reactions?**

Radiographic contrast agents (iodine-based) cause most anaphylactoid reactions.

○ **For how long should a patient with a generalized anaphylactic reaction be observed?**

24 hours. Recurrence and delayed reactions are possible. Patients should be treated with oral antihistamines and corticosteroids for at least 72 hours.

○ **A rheumatoid arthritis (RA) patient presenting with painful speaking or swallowing, hoarseness, or stridor could have what type of complication?**

Involvement of the paired cricoarytenoid joints. These may become fixed in the closed position, resulting in airway compromise.

○ **What percentage of patients with systemic lupus erythematosus (SLE) will develop signs and symptoms of pleurisy during the course of their disease?**

Approximately half. Pleurisy is also common in RA, but is often asymptomatic. All pulmonary effusions in patients with rheumatic disease require thoracentesis to distinguish from infectious processes.

○ **Myocardial infarction can be related to which two rheumatic diseases?**

Kawasaki disease and polyarteritis nodosa.

○ **A patient presents with fever, acute polyarthritis, or migratory arthritis a few weeks after a bout of Streptococcal pharyngitis; they should be evaluated for what disease?**

Rheumatic fever. Approximately 30% will have subcutaneous nodules, erythema marginatum, or chorea.

○ **What is the drug of choice for the fever and arthritis of rheumatic fever?**

Salicylates and bedrest until signs and symptoms return to normal.

○ **What clinical sign do the following often have in common: rheumatic fever, bacterial endocarditis, Schonlein-Henoch purpura, prodromal pulmonary Mycoplasma, or fungal infections?**

Migratory arthritis.

○ **What pathological process should be considered in a patient treated with steroids, who presents with weakness, depression, fatigue, and postural dizziness?**

Adrenal insufficiency. Treatment consists of stress steroids—dexamethasone is preferred because it does not interfere with testing of adrenal steroids levels.

○ **Name a common complication of SLE, RA, and JRA.**

Pericarditis.

○ **Polymyalgia rheumatica coexists in 10–30% of patients with which disease affecting the vascular system?**

Temporal arteritis.

○ **What is the *most common* pathogen found in osteomyelitis and septic arthritis of the foot?**

Pseudomonas.

○ **How does the time course of the onset of joint pain help differentiate between gout and pseudogout?**

Patients with gout develop joint pain over a few hours, while pseudogout usually evolves over a day.

○ **What is the first priority in the workup of a patient suspected of having gout?**

Exclusion of septic arthritis.

○ **How may an olecranon bursitis be differentiated from arthritis of the elbow?**

Bursitis will not affect pronation or supination.

○ **What are the two *most common* causes of fatal anaphylaxis?**

(1) Drug reactions, 95% to penicillin. Parenteral most dangerous. 300 people/y.

(2) Hymenoptera stings. 100 people/y.

○ **Food mediated hypersensitivity reactions are due to what component of the immune system?**

IgE. Dairy products, nuts, and eggs are the most common.

○ **When do the clinical manifestations of a drug allergy reaction usually become apparent?**

The first or second week following administration of the drug.

○ **Generalized malaise, fever, arthralgias, and urticaria are common to what type of allergic reaction?**

Drug allergy. Allergic reactions to drugs may involve any or all of the four types of hypersensitivity reactions.

○ **How long after exposure to an allergen does anaphylaxis occur?**

Between 1 second and 1 hour of exposure.

○ **How long should a patient with a generalized anaphylactic reaction be observed?**

For at least 24 hours.

○ **What joint is most commonly affected with gout?**

The great toe metatarsal phalangeal joint.

○ **What hypersensitivity skin rashes are noted with phenytoin use?**

Lupus-like and Stevens-Johnson syndrome.

○ **How does obesity affect the development of osteoarthritis?**

Osteoarthritis is a degenerative joint disease caused by the wear and tear on weight bearing joints. Obesity increases this wear and tear, and can worsen osteoarthritis.

○ **A butterfly rash across the bridge of the nose is a characteristic sign of what connective tissue disorder?**

Systemic lupus erythematosus (SLE).

○ **What is the *most common* allergic reaction to penicillin?**

Rash.

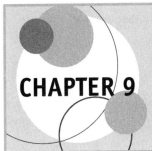

CHAPTER 9

Genitourinary/Renal Pearls

○ **A 50-year-old female is admitted to the medsurg floor with acute glomerulonephritis (GN). Describe findings in patients with GN.**

Hematuria

Proteinuria

Oliguria or anuria

Edema

Hypertension

○ **Acute tubular necrosis (ATN) resulting from two different mechanisms is the *most common* cause of intrinsic renal failure. Name the two mechanisms.**

Ischemic injury and nephrotoxic agents.

○ **Name some common drugs/substances that can contribute to renal failure.**

Aminoglycosides, NSAIDs, contrast agents (radiology tests such as CT contrast dye, cardiac catheterization, etc.), myoglobin (from compartment syndrome, massive muscle trauma).

○ **What are the risk factors for subclinical pyelonephritis?**

Those are the things that make someone more likely to have it. They include multiple prior UTIs, longer duration of UTIs, recent pyelonephritis, diabetes, anatomic abnormalities, partial obstruction (ureterolithiasis or scarred/damaged ureters), immunocompromised patients and those who are indigent/limited access to medical care.

○ **Contrast the pain associated with epididymitis to that of prostatitis.**

Epididymitis: Pain begins in scrotum or groin, involves significant tenderness and swelling of the involved testicle, pain radiates along spermatic cord, often intensifies quickly after onset, may be associated with dysuria, and may be relieved by scrotal elevation.

Prostatitis: Acute prostatitis is associated with more urinary frequency, dysuria and urgency, bladder outlet obstruction and retention, low back and perineal area pain associated with fever and chills, and with arthralgias and myalgias.

Patients with either of these disorders may become toxic, febrile, and require admission.

○ **T/F: Testicular torsion often occurs after exertion or during sleep.**

True.

○   **T/F: About 40% of patients with testicular torsion have a history of a similar pain that resolved spontaneously.**

True.

○   **With what condition is the "blue dot" sign associated?**

Torsion of the testicular appendage (lower pole of the testicle, causing pain and focal tenderness and a blue-colored appearance through the thin-skinned scrotum).

○   **What is the eponym for idiopathic scrotal gangrene?**

Fournier's gangrene. This is a life-threatening infection that spreads rapidly throughout the perineum, and unless antibiotics and surgery are instituted soon, the patient is at risk of severe complications and death.

○   **A penile fracture is actually a tear of the tunica albuginea and requires surgery to appose the ends of the tunica and to evacuate the hematoma. Is a retrograde urethrogram necessary in the evaluation of a patient with this injury?**

Yes, though uncommon, the urethra can be disrupted.

○   **What are most renal calculi made out of?**

70% of renal calculi are composed of calcium oxalate.

○   **About what percentage of renal stones are radiopaque (can actually see on a plain x-ray of the kidneys/ureter/bladder)?**

90%. The other 10% are radiolucent (unable to see on plain x-ray).

○   **About what percentage of renal calculi will pass spontaneously?**

90%. If the kidney stone is 5 mm or larger in size, it is much less likely to pass and will likely need surgery (cystoscopy with instrumentation/basket-retrieval by a urology doctor).

○   **What is the most commonly used procedure to treat urinary calcili that reside in the kidneys?**

Extracorporeal shock wave lithotripsy. Ultrasononic shock waves pulverize the calculi into many small fragments that later pass through the urinary tract over the next few weeks to months.

○   **What are some causes of false-positive hematuria?**

Food coloring, beets, paprika, rifampin, phenothiazines, Dilantin, myoglobin, or menstruation.

○   **What is the *most common* cause of hematuria?**

Lesions of the bladder or lower urinary tract. When hematuria originates in a kidney, the probable causes are polycystic kidney disease and nephropathy. Anyone with hematuria should have its source identified. A repeat or followup urinalysis should be performed. Cancer or other serious problems should be ruled out.

○   **What is the post void residual volume that suggests urinary retention?**

A volume greater than 75 cc. This places the patient at increased risk for UTIs.

○ **What is the definition of oliguria?**

A urine output of less than 500 ml/day, or less than 30 cc/hour.

○ **What is the definition of anuria?**

Urine output of less than 100 ml/day.

○ **What are the risk factors for pyelonephritis?**

Multiple prior UTIs, longer duration of symptoms, recent pyelonephritis, diabetes, and anatomic abnormalities. Immunocompromised patients and indigents are also at greater risk.

○ **What is the *most common* cause of chronic renal failure?**

NIDDM. Noninsulin dependent diabetes mellitus. Chronic hypertension is another common cause.

○ **When are the symptoms related to renal insufficiency displayed?**

When 90% of the nephrons have been destroyed. Hypertension, diabetes mellitus, glomerulonephritis, polycystic kidney disease, tubulointerstitial disease, and obstructive uropathy are all causes of chronic renal failure.

○ **What are the three different categories of acute renal failure?**

Prerenal, intrinsic, and postrenal.

○ **What are the causes of prerenal failure, or prerenal azotemia?**

Hypovolemia, dehydration, hemorrhage, burns, AMI, arrhythmia, vascular failure, sepsis, anaphylaxis, acidosis, or renal artery occlusion.

○ **What are the causes of intrarenal (intrinsic) failure?**

Acute tubular necrosis (ATN, causing 80–90%), resulting from either an ischemic injury or a nephrotoxic agent. Less frequent causes of intrinsic renal failure (10–20%) include vasculitis, malignant hypertension, allergic interstitial nephritis, acute glomerulonephritis, nephrotoxic drugs or chemicals (antibiotics, anticancer, fluorinated anesthetic, heavy metal, or radiographic contrast dye).

○ **What are the causes of postrenal failure?**

This occurs when urine flow is obstructed or venous blood flow from the kidney is obstructed. Causes include: ureter compression, strictures, or obstruction; renal calculi/kidney stones, benign prostatic hyperplasia (BPH), prostate cancer, congenital malformation, and bilateral renal vein thrombosis. Many of these conditions are reversible.

○ **What are the three phases of acute renal failure?**

An oliguric or anuric phase, a diuretic phase, and a recovery phase. The oliguric phase produces a BUN level of 25–30 mg/dl, creatinin level of 1.5–2, urine output less than 400 cc/day, or aneuria. The diuretic phases cause a gradual return of renal function, but the large amount of urine produced may be associated with a large loss of sodium, potassium and magnesium, with continued elevated BUN and creatinine. The recovery phase continues with gradual return of BUN and creatinine to normal.

○ **A 58-year-old female is admitted to medsurg that has renal failure. She is on telemetry and ventricular tachycardia is noted. You immediately check the patient and she is unresponsive with no pulse. What medications and treatments are used to treat a patient with hyperkalemia who develops cardiopulmonary arrest?**

An easy way to remember this is "C-BIG-K-Drop."

C = calcium chloride (central line) or calcium gluconate (peripheral IV).

B = bicarbonate (sodium bicarbonate rapid IV push).

I = insulin (regular, 10 units IV push).

G = glucose (push 1 amp/50 cc of D-50).

K = kaexalate (oral or rectal, polystyrene sulfonate, of limited use in full arrest).

D = dialysis (hyperkalemic renal patients benefit from dialysis at appropriate times).

○ **What are the three types of dialysis used to treat acute renal failure?**

Peritoneal dialysis, hemodialysis, and CRRT (continuous renal replacement therapy). Peritoneal dialysis has the advantage of allowing home use, and is more gentle on the cardiovascular system for those with cardiac disease, and because there is no heparinization required it can be used for patients with GI bleeding, cerebral bleeds, or recent surgery. Hemodialysis is used for patients with more severe renal disease, fluid overload, or hyperkalemia because it removes wastes and fluids more rapidly than peritoneal dialysis. If the patient had recent abdomen surgery or adhesions, then peritoneal dialysis may be contraindicated. CRRT is used for critically ill patients who cannot tolerate peritoneal or hemodialysis due to poor hemodyanmic stability, as it is used 24 hours a day overall several days to slowly remove wastes.

○ **A 46-year-old diabetic with end stage renal disease is admitted to the floor. Describe treatment options for advanced chronic renal disease.**

End-stage renal disease occurs when the glomerular filtration rate (GFR) falls below 100 ml/minute or less than 10–15% below the normal rate, then the patient requires long-term dialysis or kidney transplantation. Special diet (low protein to decrease nitrogen load, high calorie, high carbohydrate), special medicines, limitation of fluid intake, activity limitations, and other measures are used to optimize treatment. These patients are relatively immunocompromised, and often develop anemia requiring medications and occasional transfusions of blood.

○ **The above patient is placed on fluid intake restriction due to volume overload. What would this likely be?**

If urine output is low and fluid overload becomes a problem, then fluid intake is often restricted to the previous day's urine output plus 500 cc for insensible losses (perspiration, moisture lost from breathing, etc.).

○ **Dietary potassium is not restricted if the renal patient has a daily urine production of more than _____ milliliters.**

1,000 ml per day urine output. The exception is if the serum potassium level is higher than 5.5 mEq/l.

○ **What is the *most common* cause of urethritis in males?**

Neisseria gonorrhea and Chlamydia trachomatis. In elderly males, the more likely cause is *E. coli* and other coloniform bacteria.

○ **What bacteria is the *most common* cause of UTIs in uncatheterized elderly patients?**

E. coli.

○ **What is the *most common* cause of nongonococcal urethritis?**

Chlamydia trachomatis. Ureaplasma urealyticum is another common cause.

○ **What is the *most common* cause of epididymitis?**

Chlamydia trachomatis.

○ **What findings mark the presentation of a patient with rapidly progressive glomerulonephritis?**

Hematuria (most common), edema (periorbital), HTN, ascites, pleural effusion, rales, and anuria.

○ **What is phimosis?**

A condition in which the foreskin cannot be retracted posterior to the glands. The preliminary treatment is performing minor surgery, making a dorsal slit in the foreskin to allow retraction. Sometimes circumcision is necessary to complete treatment.

○ **What is paraphimosis?**

A condition in which the foreskin is retracted posterior to the glands and cannot be advanced over the glands. This may cause severe swelling and possible ischemia of the glans penis and therefore in severe cases is a surgical emergency.

○ **What are the causes of priapism?**

Prolonged sex, leukemia, sickle cell trait and disease, blood dyscrasias, pelvic hematoma or neoplasm, syphilis, urethritis, and drugs including phenothiazines, prazosin, tolbutamide, anticoagulants, and corticosteroids.

○ **Why would you be concerned if a quadriplegic suddenly develops a severe headache?**

It is a symptom of autonomic dysreflexia. Bladder distention is one of the most common causes. The nurse should assess for this, as well as other causes including rectal impaction or distension, stimulation of the perineum, sacral ulcers, and other diseases causing pain or nerve stimulation.

○ **What are some of the symptoms of disequilibrium syndrome in a patient with chronic renal failure?**

Hypertension, headache, confusion, nausea, and vomiting.

○ **What is the physiological reason for disequilibrium syndrome?**

During dialysis, excess solutes are cleared from the blood at a faster pace than they can diffuse from the body's cells into the circulatory system.

○ **What is a common and potentially dangerous complication of peritoneal dialysis?**

Peritonitis.

○ **What is the purpose of giving aluminum hydroxide (Amphojel) to a patient with chronic renal failure?**

It binds phosphates in foods and is administered with or immediately after meals.

○ **Why are patients with chronic renal failure often nauseated?**

The presence of retained waste products in the body often causes nausea. Nitrogen wastes, amino acids, BUN, and other waste products build up and cause lethargy, nausea, and generalized malaise.

○   **Acute renal failure caused by an obstruction in the urinary tract would be what category of renal failure?**

Postrenal.

○   **Why do patients with chronic renal failure often have dry itchy skin?**

Uremia causes this due to the retention of nitrogenous wastes, which leads to uric acid crystals and other nitrogen wastes to build up on the skin, sometimes causing a "uremic frost" appearance.

○   **What should be a priority nursing goal for a patient with renal calculi?**

Relieve the patient's pain and control the nausea/vomiting with medications.

○   **Where is the best place to secure a Foley catheter to prevent irritation?**

To the upper inner thigh. The male patient may also have the Foley secured to his abdomen.

○   **What are some of the common symptoms of cystitis?**

Dysuria, hematuria, burning upon urination, urgency, and frequency.

○   **What serum blood test is the best indicator of renal function?**

Serum creatinine. The creatinine clearance test would be an accurate indicator also.

○   **What symptoms would you expect to find if peritonitis was present in a patient on continuous ambulatory peritoneal dialysis (CAPD)?**

Cloudy dialysate fluid returns, hyperactive bowel sounds, abdominal pain, and fever.

○   **What is the purpose of phenazopyridine (Pyridium) in the treatment of cystitis?**

It is used as a local analgesic that numbs the bladder that relieves some of the discomfort associated with cystitis.

○   **What side effect of phenazopyridine (Pyridium) should a patient be made aware of?**

Bright red-orange urine results and is no cause for alarm. Patients should be warned that their urine will stain underwear and contact lenses orange.

○   **What is the best way to obtain a urine specimen from a patient with a Foley catheter?**

Ideally the best way is to remove the Foley catheter, and replace it with a new catheter, and send urine specimens from the new collection system. Chronic indwelling Foley catheters nearly always are infected; the question is whether or not there is a clinically important bladder or renal infection. If the Foley cannot be replaced, then a sterile aspiration of the tube as proximal possible should be done. Cleanse access port with alcohol and insert needless needle and 20 cc syringe in port. Withdraw at least 15 cc for a UA and C&S.

○   **You insert a Foley catheter into a patient with an overdistended bladder, but partially clamp the tubing to allow the urine to drain at a slow rate. Why?**

Rapidly emptying an overdistended bladder may cause shock and hypotension due to the rapid decrease in pressure in the abdominal viscera. You should only remove up to 1000 cc of urine to prevent bladder spasms, wait 10–15 minutes and then remove the rest of the urine.

○ **A urinalysis report indicates the presence of red blood cells and white blood cells. What is the most likely cause?**

Urinary tract infection.

○ **What is the *most common* bacterial infections in all patients?**

UTI. UTIs increase in frequency with age, and are more common in women.

○ **A 37-year-old female is admitted with a fever of 103 F, nausea, vomiting, flank pain and CVA tenderness, tachycardia, and chills. She recently returned from her honeymoon. Her diagnosis most likely is _____?**

Acute pyelonephritis.

○ **A 65-year-old male is admitted for presumed kidney stone due to his severe left flank pain and hematuria. He becomes hypotensive, and complaints of worse flank pain. You check the chart and see that he has not had his CT scan to diagnose the kidney stone. Other possible causes of this patient's symptoms include what?**

Abdominal aortic aneurysm, or AAA (triple-A). In 25% of patients with a leaking or dissecting abdominal aortic aneurysm, there will be hematuria found due to the retroperitoneal bleeding near the kidneys and ureter that cause hematuria, leading the medical staff to suspect a kidney stone instead of life-threatening causes.

○ **In males, what is the *most common* symptom that causes patients to seek treatment for gonorrhea?**

Painful urination and mucopurulent discharge.

○ **How should you assess for a distended bladder?**

A distended bladder will produce an uncomfortable rounded swelling in the lower abdomen above the symphysis pubis.

○ **What is the easiest method and most effective way to prevent a urinary tract infection in a patient with a spinal cord injury?**

Drink at least 2000 ml/day of fluid.

○ **In a patient who cannot void, the first nursing action should be?**

Assess the bladder by palpation. Increasingly bedside or urology ultrasound machines are available for bladder measurement by nursing staff.

○ **What is a chancre?**

A painless ulcerative lesion that develops during the primary stage of syphilis.

○ **What is the most prevalent sexually transmitted disease in the United States?**

Chlamydia.

○ **What are the signs and symptoms of secondary syphilis?**

Enlarged lymph nodes, alopecia, erosions of the oral mucosa, and a rash on the palms and soles.

○ **What are the characteristics of nephrotic syndrome?**

Proteinuria, hypoalbuminemia, edema, and ascites.

○ **How can you tell if a dialysis shunt is functioning properly?**

A thrill (vibration) can be palpated or a bruit can be auscultated with a stethoscope.

○ **What is the normal BUN value?**

10–20 mg/dL.

○ **What should be done with the urine of a patient with suspected renal or urethral calculi?**

Strain for calculi. The patient should be given instructions to use a metal screen strainer to urinate in or pour collected urine through in attempts to collect and analyze the kidney stone, in hopes of modifying diet or other factors to prevent future stones.

○ **What is the treatment for gonorrhea?**

Ceftriaxone 125 mg IM, or a single oral tablet of an approved flouroquinolone, plus treatment for Chlamydia (use doxycycline or azithromycin). The latter is given because half of all patients infected with gonorrhea are simultaneously infected with Chlamydia. Any patients who have become infected in Europe or by gay men should not be given fluoroquinolones due to increasing resistance.

○ **What is the *most common* medical complication of pregnancy?**

Urinary tract infections.

○ **Torsion of the testicles is *most common* in what age group?**

Adolescents. Any male with significant testicle pain should be fully assessed and have torsion ruled out by Doppler ultrasound, nuclear medicine perfusion testing, or surgery. Significant torsion is usually accompanied by nausea and vomiting and severe pain.

○ **Testicular torsion is *most common* in which age group?**

In 14 year olds. Two-thirds of the cases occur in the second decade. The next most common group is newborns.

○ **What is the definitive treatment for testicular torsion?**

Surgery. Bilateral orchiopexy in which the testes are surgically attached to the scrotum.

○ **Besides the white blood cell count, what results from a urinalysis would indicate a UTI?**

Protein, a pH greater than 8, leukocyte esterase, and nitrite.

○ **What is nephrotic syndrome?**

It is an altered glomerular permeability that results in the excretion of large amount of protein in the urine.

○ **How is a hydrocele differentiated from an inguinal hernia?**

A hydrocele can be transilluminated (using a small flashlight or otoscope, the light can be easily seen shining through the hydrocele because it is basically a clear fluid collection). A hernia cannot because of the presence of intestines (do not transmit light) in the scrotal sac.

○ **A client with glomerulonephritis has an elevated blood pressure. What should you be assessing for?**

Symptoms of hypertensive encephalopathy.

○ **A patient with glomerulonephritis is oliguric but has been placed on a fluid restriction. Why?**

Because the urine output is lower. In glomerulonephritis, the kidneys are no longer functioning normally and fluid that is taken in is retained. Edema, weight gain, and elevated blood pressure could result from the retention of fluids.

○ **What is the major risk factor associated with peritoneal dialysis?**

Peritonitis.

○ **What is the pathophysiology of nephrotic syndrome?**

Altered glomerular permeability resulting in the excretion of a large amount of protein in the urine.

○ **What are the indications of an infection at the (CAPD) catheter exit site?**

Redness, pain, tenderness, swelling, and drainage.

○ **When peritonitis is present, what will the dialysate fluid look like?**

Cloudy due to the large number of bacteria, fibrin, and white blood cells. A cell count, Gram stain, and culture will differentiate the diagnosis further.

○ **A pleasant 64-year-old male is admitted to the medsurg floor for mild chest pain. He is pain free, but relates that he has significant difficulty urinating for the past month. He has dull back pain also for the past few weeks, and it is getting worse. What diagnosis should be ruled out and how is this best accomplished?**

Prostate cancer. Any change in bowel or bladder habits should be looked into carefully by the medical team. This patient may have prostate cancer with metastatic disease to his lower spine. An evaluation would include a careful history and physical exam, including rectal exam with prostate palpation, hemocult stool, urinalysis, PSA (prostate-specific antigen, elevated in prostate cancer and significant hypertrophy), and possible prostate ultrasound and biopsy. If cancer or BPH (benign prostatic hypertrophy) is discovered, then further treatment would be indicated.

CHAPTER 10

Resuscitation and Shock Pearls

○ **About what percentage of patients who undergo full cardiopulmonary arrest, undergo cardiac resuscitation, recover and are neurologically intact?**

10%.

○ **About what percentage of patients who undergo cardiac resuscitation survive, but are not functionally and neurologically intact?**

25%.

○ **About what percentage of patients in trauma-related full arrest survive?**

0.1%; only one in a thousand survive traumatic full arrest.

○ **When administering CPR per 2005 AHA guidelines, what is the ventilation to compression ratio for one rescuer?**

The new compression to ventilation ratio is 30:2, which is done until the airway is secured with an advanced airway (ET or other tube). The chest compression rate is 100 per minute "fast and hard" with depth of compressions 1.5–2 inches deep. When an advanced airway is placed, then chest compression should be continued with minimal to no interruptions, while the ventilations are independently interposed at a rate of 8–10 ventilations per minute (one breath every 6–8 seconds). Each rescue breath should be given over 1 second to make the chest rise, and not breaths that are too large or forceful. For the "witnessed arrest," as soon as a defibrillator or AED is available, the cardiac rhythm should be assessed. If the patient is noted to be in VF or pulseless V-tach, a singe shock of 360 J (monophasic defibrillator) or appropriate setting for biphasic defibrillator) should be performed and immediately after this, chest compressions should be resumed without checking for a pulse. If the patient has an "unwitnessed arrest" or arrives at the hospital with prior collapse unwitnessed by staff, then CPR should be performed for at least 2 minutes (five cycles of 30:2 compressions to ventilations) BEFORE attempting defibrillation. If there is evidence of spontaneous return of circulation, CPR may be stopped. Otherwise, CPR should be continued for the next 2 minutes or approximately five cycles of CPR. Reassessment should then occur. Resuscitators should also change every 2 minutes if adequate help is available, to ensure compressions are delivered appropriately.

○ **What is the ventilation to compression ratio for two rescuers?**

Laypersons and single rescuers should always use the same 30:2 compression-to-ventilation ratio for all victims of all ages. Health care providers (HCPs) are to use 30:2 ratio for all adults (1 or 2 rescuers), but in children and infants HCPs are to use 15:2 compression-to-ventilation ratio if there are 2 HCP rescuers present.

○ **What is the *most common* source of sepsis in the elderly?**

Respiratory > urinary > intra-abdominal.

○   **How does pallor appear in a black patient?**

The skin is yellow/brown or gray due to the loss of the underlying red tones. The conjunctiva will appear pale.

○   **A patient is found in the medsurg bed with a decreased level of consciousness, a BP of 45/15, shallow respirations, and ventricular tachycardia on the monitor. What should you do first?**

Prepare to defibrillate this unstable patient and call for help in resuscitation. Pulses should be confirmed and vital signs checked frequently. Institute CPR when appropriate.

○   **After a patient is brought back to a normal sinus rhythm following defibrillation, what medication will most likely be ordered?**

IV lidocaine or amiodarone bolus and an infusion.

○   **A 70-year-old man visiting his wife in the hospital suddenly loses consciousness and collapses. What should be your first action?**

Ensure scene safety and personal protective equipment, then the first step in basic life support is to assess the level of consciousness and attempt to arouse the patient, shouting, "Are you OK?" and call out the patient's name.

○   **After you determine the patient to be unresponsive, what is your next step?**

Call for help and then begin assessing the "ABCs": airway, breathing, and circulation. The airway, breathing and circulation (pulse) "ABCs" should be rapidly assessed, and if an abnormal or absent pulse is found, then rapid assessment with an AED or other defibrillator should be performed. Defibrillation or cardioversion, CPR, and ACLS should then be provided per protocol.

○   **Above what level of oxygen concentration is there an increased risk for causing oxygen toxicity?**

40%. Note that room air oxygen concentration is approximately 21%, and is lower at higher altitude.

○   **What conclusion can be drawn from a PaO_2 level of 50 in a client that exhibits no signs or symptoms of hypoxia?**

The arterial blood gas is not truly arterial.

○   **What is an early behavioral sign of hypoxia?**

Anxiety and any change in level of consciousness.

○   **Describe some of the common signs of cardiogenic shock.**

Low blood pressure, oliguria, crackles (rales) in the lungs, rapid and weak pulse, and diminished blood flow to the brain (altered mental status, seizures).

○   **What is the correct compression rate for one man and two man CPR in an adult?**

100 per minute.

○   **What is the correct ventilation rate during rescue breathing without chest compressions for adults? What is the correct rate for infants and children?**

The rescue breathing without chest compressions rate for adults is 10–12 breaths/min, and for children and infants is 12–20 breaths/min.

○ **What is the correct rescue breath rate for CPR with an advanced airway in adults, children, and infants?**

8–10 breaths/min (approx 1 breath every 6–8 seconds).

○ **What are some of the toxic effects of lidocaine?**

Confusion, dizziness, tremors, blurred vision, tinnitus, numbness and tingling of the extremities, hypotension, convulsions, and coma.

○ **What is the mechanism of action of lidocaine upon heart tissue?**

It decreases automaticity of the His-purkinje fibers and raises the stimulation threshold in the ventricles.

○ **You find a patient that is unconscious. What should you do first?**

Scene safety and PPE. Assess level of consciousness by shaking gently and calling to the patient attempting to arouse. If the patient does not respond, then assess the ABCs and provide respiratory support as best possible.

○ **What is the proper hand technique for chest compressions in an infant?**

Using two fingertips pressed at the breastbone just below the nipple line. For healthcare providers, an additional method is placing thumbs together on the sternum, one finger's width below the nipple line, and encompassing the chest with the other fingers and hands, then compressing the chest during CPR.

○ **Which is one of the earliest signs of sepsis?**

Respiratory alkalosis on an ABG.

○ **How should you position a patient before beginning CPR?**

On a firm surface, on his back.

○ **A patient is hyperventilating and blood gases are drawn. What results would you expect to see?**

Normal pO_2, decreased pCO_2, increased pH: Respiratory alkalosis.

○ **What is the primary physiological alteration that occurs with shock?**

Inadequate tissue perfusion.

○ **If the chest wall fails to rise during rescue breathing, what could be the cause?**

Airway obstruction, caused by the tongue or a foreign body, or the head not in the proper position.

○ **When is it acceptable to discontinue CPR?**

When the rescuer is exhausted, the physician orders it to be discontinued, or there is not another rescuer available to continue CPR, or the family delivers an advance directive and the EMS protocols allow termination of CPR by that level of EMS crew.

○ **What is the *most common* cause of death following a myocardial infarction?**

Cardiac dysrhythmias.

○   **What is the death rate for patients with an acute myocardial infarction who are treated in the hospital?**

7%.

○   **What is the death rate for patients with an acute myocardial infarction who are accidentally or unintentionally discharged home?**

14%.

○   **What is the best method of evaluating whether oxygen therapy is effective for a patient?**

Arterial blood gases.

○   **What is cardiogenic shock?**

Cardiac output is decreased because of inadequate myocardial contractility leading to inadequate tissue perfusion.

○   **How can you determine if the fluid replacement therapy administered to a dehydrated patient was effective?**

The urine output is the most sensitive indicator of hydration. It should amount to 30 cc per hour minimum for adequate hydration.

○   **In the absence of renal or cardiac problems, what should be the normal urine output in a patient who is adequately hydrated?**

30–35 ml/hour or greater.

○   **During rescue breathing in CPR, how is the patient able to exhale?**

Passive relaxation of the chest will force air out naturally.

○   **What purpose does dopamine hydrochloride serve in the treatment of cardiogenic shock?**

It increases myocardial contractility, thus increasing cardiac output.

○   **In low doses, how does dopamine affect the kidneys?**

It dilates the renal arteries increasing renal perfusion.

○   **What nursing assessment is essential during the administration of dopamine?**

Monitoring blood pressure closely.

○   **What is the reason for administering epinephrine to a patient during CPR?**

It causes vasoconstriction of the peripheral blood flow and increases systemic vascular resistance, increasing venous return to the heart. It also stimulates the adrenergic receptors of the heart and can increase impulse conduction, thus stimulating some cardiac activity.

○   **What is the preferred position for a patient who is hypovolemic?**

Flat, with the legs elevated as long as the lung sounds are clear and there is no spinal column compromise or large leg bone fracture.

○ **What should be the depth of compressions in an adult when performing CPR?**

$1\frac{1}{2}''$–$2''$ or enough to provide a strong perfusing pulse.

○ **What is considered the maximum amount of time that a person can be pulseless, without CPR, and not experience brain damage?**

4–6 minutes.

○ **What age groups are at risk for septic shock due to infection?**

The very young and the elderly.

○ **What common invasive device is a frequent cause of sepsis in the elderly?**

The Foley catheter.

○ **You determine that a patient is breathless and pulseless. After calling for help and positioning him on his back, what should you do next?**

Open the airway and administer two breaths.

○ **What are some of the signs of early septic shock?**

Warm flushed skin, confusion, restlessness, tachycardia, and tachypnea.

○ **As septic shock progresses, how does the skin exam change?**

The skin becomes cool and clammy.

○ **During CPR in adults, what artery should be used to check the pulse?**

Carotid.

○ **If cardiac compressions are performed inappropriately, what organ is in danger of being damaged?**

The liver.

○ **How do you calculate pulse pressure?**

Systolic pressure minus diastolic pressure.

○ **What are the typical criteria for brain death (these may vary from state to state)?**

Unresponsiveness to painful stimuli, absence of spontaneous respiration or muscle movement, and loss of brainstem function (as evidenced by fixed, dilated pupils and absence of reflexes, and a flat electroencephalogram).

○ **What result can occur from using a blood pressure cuff that is too wide?**

A falsely decreased blood pressure reading may be obtained.

○ **What is the drug of choice for reducing premature ventricular contractions?**

Lidocaine hydrochloride or amiodarone according to the AHA.

○   **What are the signs and symptoms of hypovolemia?**

Rapid weak pulse, low blood pressure, cool clammy skin, shallow respirations, oliguria or anuria, and lethargy.

○   **When using one hand to ventilate an adult patient with an Ambu bag, how many ccs of air are delivered?**

400 cc.

○   **When using two hands to ventilate with an Ambu bag, how much air can be delivered?**

1,000 cc of air.

○   **What may hypotension indicate in a patient with an MI?**

Cardiogenic shock in most cases. Rarely it can be from pericardial tamponade.

○   **Describe arterial bleeding.**

Bright red, flows rapidly, and spurts with each heartbeat.

○   **What is pulsus alternans?**

A regular pulse rhythm with an alternation of weak and strong beats. It occurs in ventricular enlargement, because the stroke volume varies with each heart beat.

○   **Define cardiac output.**

The volume of blood ejected from the heart per minute. It is expressed as liters per minute. It is equal to the heart rate multiplied by the stroke volume. So if there are 70 beats per minute, and 70 ml blood is ejected with each beat of the heart, the cardiac output is 4,900 ml/minute. This value is typical for an average adult at rest, although cardiac output may reach up to 30 l/minute during extreme exercise. When cardiac output increases in a healthy but untrained individual, most of the increase can be attributed to increase in heart rate. Change of posture, increased sympathetic nervous system activity, and decreased parasympathetic nervous system activity can also increase cardiac output. Heart rate can vary by a factor of approximately 3, between 60 and 180 beats per minute, while stroke volume can vary between 70 and 120 ml, a factor of only 1.7.

○   **Define stroke volume.**

The volume of blood ejected from the heart during systole, usually in an adult ranges from 70–120 ml with each heart contraction (stroke).

○   **What is the *most common* cause of septic shock?**

Gram-negative bacteria such as *E. coli, Klebsiella pneumonia,* and *K. pseudomonas.*

○   **What is the *most common* cause of airway obstruction in an unconscious patient?**

The tongue.

○   **What is capillary refill time?**

The amount of time required for color to return to the nail beds after application of slight pressure which causes blanching, normally less 3 seconds. In patients with low blood pressure or sometimes cold fingers/skin, this will be delayed longer than 3 seconds.

○   **What is the treatment of choice for patients with pulseless ventricular tachycardia?**

Defibrillation (unsynchronized).

○   **About what percentage of normal *coronary blood* flow is achieved during CPR?**

5%.

○   **About what percentage of normal *cardiac output* is achieved during CPR?**

20–25%.

○   **What is the currently favored theory explaining how CPR works?**

The thoracic pump theory—that blood flow is induced by a pressure gradient between the intrathoracic and extrathoracic compartments.

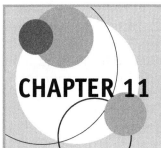

CHAPTER 11

Hematology/Oncology Pearls

○ **An adult patient receives a major head injury. He also suffers from classic hemophilia, what medical treatment should be given?**

Give Factor VIII 50 U/kg.

○ **What lab abnormalities does Disseminated Intravascular Coagulation (DIC) cause?**

Increased PT, elevated fibrin split products, decreased fibrinogen and thrombocytopenia.

○ **What type of hemophilia results from a deficiency of factor 9 is sex linked and has a positive family history?**

Christmas disease or hemophilia B.

○ **What type of hemophilia has a factor 8 deficiency is sex linked and may present without a family history?**

Classic hemophilia. Also called hemophilia A, about 1/2 have a family hx.

○ **What type of hemophilia is autosomal dominant and has a deficiency in factor 8?**

von Willebrand's.

○ **What are the two *most common* tumors causing ischemic dysfunction of the spinal cord?**

Lymphoma and multiple myeloma.

○ **What is the most effective way to control the bleeding induced by warfarin therapy?**

Fresh frozen plasma provides fast response. Also give vitamin K, intramuscularly. May want to check test dose first.

○ **What laboratory abnormalities would be expected in a patient with platelet dysfunction?**

Abnormal bleeding time with normal PT, normal PTT and normal platelet count. NSAIDs are a common cause of abnormal platelet function.

○ **What are the common features of thrombocytopenic purpura?**

Thrombocytopenia, microangiopathic hemolytic anemia, fever, renal failure, and fluctuating neurologic symptoms. Coagulation studies are typically normal.

○ **What clotting study is typically abnormal with thrombocytopenia?**

Bleeding time.

Usually thrombocytopenia is an acquired disorder secondary to infections, drugs or autoimmune disease. As platelets are not involved in the intrinsic or extrinsic clotting pathways, both PT and PTT remain normal.

○ **Name four conditions that may cause reactive thrombocytosis.**

Iron deficiency, postsplenectomy, malignancy, and infection.

○ **A cancer patient presents with a history of constipation, decreased mental status, and back pain. What electrolyte imbalance could be present?**

Hypercalcemia. *Remember:* the signs and symptoms of hypercalcemia include nausea, vomiting, anorexia, constipation, polyuria, hypertension, and decreased mentation.

○ **What factors are deficient in classic hemophilia, Christmas disease, and von Willebrand's disease, respectively?**

Classic hemophilia—Factor VIII.
Christmas disease—Factor IX.
von Willebrand's disease—Factor VIIIc + von Willebrand's cofactor.

○ **Which pathway involves factors VIII and IX?**

Intrinsic pathway.

○ **What effect does deficiency of factors VIII and IX have on PT and on PTT?**

Deficiency leads to increase in PTT.

○ **How may hemophilia A be clinically distinguished from hemophilia B?**

Hemophilia A is not clinically distinguishable from Christmas disease (hemophilia B).

○ **Which blood product is given when the coagulation abnormality is unknown?**

Fresh frozen plasma (FFP).

○ **What agent can be used for treating mild hemophilia A and von Willebrand's disease type 1?**

D-amino-8, D-arginine vasopressin (DDAVP) induces a rapid rise in factor VIII levels.

○ **Major cause of death in hemophiliacs?**

Blood component infections (HIV).

○ **Which drug reverses heparin?**

Protamine sulfate.

○ **Which types of blood loss are indicative of a bleeding disorder?**

Spontaneous bleeding from many sites, bleeding from nontraumatic sites, delayed bleeding several hours after trauma, and bleeding into deep tissues or joints.

○ **What common drugs may cause patients to acquire a bleeding disorder?**

Ethanol, salicylates, NSAIDs, warfarin, and antibiotics.

○ **Below what platelet count is spontaneous hemorrhage likely to occur?**

$<10,000/mm^3$.

○ **How can an overdose of warfarin be medically treated? What are the advantages and disadvantages of each treatment?**

Treatment depends on the severity of symptoms, not the degree of prolongation of the prothrombin time (PT). If there are no signs of bleeding, temporary discontinuation may be all that is necessary; if bleeding is present, treatment can be initiated with fresh frozen plasma (FFP) or vitamin K.

Advantages of FFP: rapid repletion of coagulation factors and control of hemorrhage. Disadvantages: volume overload, possible viral transmission.

Advantages of Vitamin K: ease of administration. Disadvantages: possible anaphylaxis when given IV; delayed onset of 12–24 hours; effects may last up to 2 weeks, making anticoagulation of the patient difficult or impossible.

○ **What are the clinical complications of DIC?**

Bleeding, thrombosis, and purpura fulminans.

○ **What three laboratory studies would be most helpful in establishing the diagnosis of DIC?**

(1) Prothrombin time—prolonged.

(2) Platelet count—usually low.

(3) Fibrinogen level—low.

○ **What types of clinical crises are seen in patients with sickle-cell disease?**

Vaso-occlusive (thrombotic), hematologic (sequestration and aplastic), and infectious crises.

○ **What are the mainstays of therapy for a patient in sickle-cell crisis?**

(1) Hydration.

(2) Analgesia.

(3) Oxygen (only beneficial if patient is hypoxic).

(4) Cardiac monitoring (if patient has history of cardiac disease or is having chest pain).

○ **A 55-year-old female is admitted preoperatively for a major operation. She appears pale, and the CBC conforms her hemoglobin to be 8.2. What are the three conditions under which the transfusion of PRBCs should be considered?**

(1) Acute hemorrhage (blood loss >1,500 ml).

(2) Surgical blood loss >2 l.

(3) Chronic anemia (Hgb <7–8 g/dl, symptomatic, or with underlying cardiopulmonary disease).

○ **What factors indicate the need for typing and cross matching of blood in an adult who is admitted emergently to a medsurg unit?**

(1) Evidence of shock from whatever cause.

(2) Known blood loss >1,000 ml.

(3) Gross GI bleeding.

(4) Hgb <10; Hct <30.

(5) Potential of going to surgery with further significant blood loss.

○ **What is the first step in treating all immediate transfusion reactions?**

Stop the transfusion.

○ **What infection carries the highest risk of transmission by blood transfusion?**

Hepatitis C.

○ **What is the only crystalloid fluid compatible with packed RBCs?**

Normal saline.

○ **What complication may arise when citrate is present in stored blood?**

Citrate binds calcium, which can induce hypocalcemia in a patient receiving the blood.

○ **What are the common presentations of a transfusion reaction?**

Myalgia, dyspnea, fever associated with hypocalcemia, hemolysis, allergic reactions, hyperkalemia, citrate toxicity, hypothermia, coagulopathies, and altered hemoglobin function.

○ **What is the *most common* transfusion reaction?**

Fever.

○ **You are ordered to start an IV on a client with a low platelet count. What special precautions should you take?**

Hold pressure on all unsuccessful venipuncture sites for 10 minutes, use a small gauge IV catheter, wrap the area with gauze to preserve skin integrity, and observe for any bleeding around the puncture site.

○ **Which lab test is used to determining the dosage of warfarin (Coumadin)?**

PT prothrombin time.

○ **What vitamin can decrease the anticoagulant effect of warfarin (Coumadin)?**

Vitamin K.

○ **What is an early symptom of laryngeal cancer?**

Hoarseness.

○ **What test is used to differentiate between sickle-cell trait and sickle-cell anemia?**

The hemoglobin electrophoresis test.

○ **What are the findings in a patient with polycythemia vera?**

Pruritus, painful fingers and toes, hyperuricemia, plethora (reddish, purple skin and mucosa), weakness, and easy fatigability.

○   **What blood type is considered the universal donor?**

Type O negative.

○   **What blood type is considered the universal recipient?**

Type AB positive.

○   **What medication is used to treat Coumadin overdose?**

Vitamin K.

○   **What are the signs and symptoms of chronic sickle-cell anemia?**

Cardiomegaly, systolic and diastolic murmurs, chronic fatigue, hepatomegaly, and tachycardia.

○   **What are the signs and symptoms of early sickle-cell anemia?**

Jaundice, bone pain, ischemic leg ulcers, pallor, joint swelling, chest pain, and an increased susceptibility to infection.

○   **What patient care measures should be implemented during a sickle-cell crisis?**

Bed rest, IV fluids, oxygen, analgesics, and a thorough documentation of fluid intake and output.

○   **How long should one unit of packed RBCs be administered?**

Over a 2–4-hour period.

○   **What gauge needle is used to administer packed RBCs or whole blood?**

16 or 18 gauge.

○   **Why must a large needle be used to administer whole blood or packed RBCs?**

To avoid RBC hemolysis.

○   **What is the mortality rate from receiving contaminated blood?**

50%.

○   **What should be done if a blood transfusion is not started within 30 minutes after the blood has been received from the blood bank?**

Return it to the blood bank. The refrigeration facilities on a typical nursing unit are inadequate for storing blood products.

○   **What commonly precipitates an aplastic crisis in a sickle-cell patient?**

Viral infections.

○   **What organs are most commonly damaged in sickle-cell patients?**

Spleen, lung, liver, kidney, skeleton, and skin.

○ **A patient presents with bluish discoloration of the gingiva. What diagnosis should you suspect?**

Chronic lead poisoning. Expect the erythrocyte protoporphyrin level to be elevated in this condition.

○ **How does sickle cell anemia affect blood cells?**

Blood cells are sickle shaped causing difficulty in moving through capillaries.

○ **What is the cause of sickle-cell disease?**

It is an autosomal recessive disorder, meaning that if both parents have the trait, then the child has a 25% chance of having the trait and a 50% chance of having the disease.

○ **What is an important basic principle that should be taught to a sickle-cell patient?**

Keep well hydrated. This will help prevent the cells from backing up in the smaller capillaries.

○ **What is the major cause of death in a patient with leukemia?**

Infection caused by the inability of the body to fight off pathogens due to the lack of mature white blood cells.

○ **What causes anemia and increased bleeding in a patient suffering from leukemia?**

The bone marrow overproduces white blood cells at the expense of producing red blood cells and platelets.

○ **Why are most hemophiliacs male?**

It is a sex linked trait passed on the X chromosome. Therefore, females need the trait to be present on both X chromosomes to have the disease, while males need only to have one. Females with the disease trait on one X chromosome are considered carriers of the disease.

○ **What is a hemarthrosis?**

Bleeding into the joints.

○ **What are some of the symptoms of a hemarthrosis?**

Pain and tenderness in the joint, and restricted movement. Continued bleeding results in a hot, swollen joint that is immobile.

○ **Why are hemophiliacs at a high risk for contracting AIDS?**

The clotting factors are derived from large pools of donated plasma, therefore the exposure is high due to many different blood donors. With the improved blood screening process and the manufacturing of synthetic factor, the risk of AIDS contraction for hemophiliacs is lower today.

○ **Why are intramuscular injections kept to a minimum for a patient with leukemia and hemophilia?**

Both are prone to abnormal bleeding, but for different reasons.

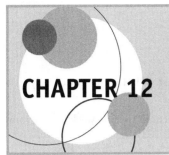

CHAPTER 12

Reproductive System Pearls

○ **Match the following terms with the appropriate definitions.**

(1) Menorrhagia
(2) Metrorrhagia (hypermenorrhea)
(3) Menometrorrhagia

(a) Bleeding between menstrual periods
(b) Excessive amount of blood or duration
(c) Excessive amount of blood at irregular frequencies

Answers: (1) (b), (2) (a), (3) (c).

○ **How much blood does a standard size pad absorb?**

20–30 ml blood.

○ **How soon after implantation can β-HCG be detected?**

2–3 days.

○ **What is the *most common* cause of toxic shock syndrome?**

The most common cause is *S. aureus*. Other causes, which are clinically similar include group A *Streptococci*, *Pseudomonas aeruginosa*, and *Streptococcus pneumoniae*.

○ **What criteria are necessary for the diagnosis of toxic shock syndrome?**

All of the following must be present: T >38.9°C (102°F), rash, systolic BP <90 and orthostasis, involvement of three organ systems (GI, renal, musculoskeletal, mucosal, hepatic, hematologic, or CNS) and negative serologic tests for such diseases as Rocky Mountain spotted fever (RMSF), hepatitis B, measles, leptospirosis, VDRL, etc.

○ **How should a patient with toxic shock syndrome be medically treated?**

FLUIDS, blood pressure support, FFP or transfusions, vaginal irrigation with iodine or saline, and antistaphylococcal penicillin or cephalosporin with anti-β-lactamase activity (nafcillin or oxacillin). Rifampin should be considered to eliminate the carrier state.

○ **A wet prep of vaginal secretions reveals clue cells. What does this indicate?**

Gardnerella vaginitis. Male partners should be treated.
     Sherlock Holmes looks for "clues" in the "Garden."

○   **What is a Bartholin's cyst?**

An obstructed Bartholin's duct that results in an abscess.

○   **A breast-feeding mother is complaining of fever, chills, and a swollen red breast. What is the most likely causative organism?**

Staphylococcus aureus is the most common cause of mastitis. Mastitis is seldom present in the first week postpartum. It is most often seen 3–4 weeks postpartum.

○   **What is the *most common* cause of vaginitis?**

Candida albicans.

○   **What gynecological infection presents with a malodorous, itchy, white to grayish, and sometimes frothy vaginal discharge?**

Trichomoniasis.

○   **Describe the presentation of a patient with Gardnerella vaginitis.**

On physical exam, a frothy, grayish-white, fishy smelling vaginal discharge is present.

○   **What does a positive Homans' sign indicate?**

The possibility that thrombophlebitis or a deep venous thrombosis is present in the lower extremities.

○   **How do you assess for Homans' sign?**

Ask the patient to stretch her legs out with the knee slightly flexed while you dorsiflex the foot. A positive sign is present when pain is felt at the back of the knee or calf.

○   **What is Goodell's sign?**

A softening of the cervix which occurs in pregnancy.

○   **What are the signs and symptoms of a chlamydial infection?**

Urinary frequency, thin white vaginal or urethral discharge, and cervical inflammation.

○   **What are the findings of premenstrual syndrome?**

Abdominal distention, backache, headache, nervousness, irritability, engorged and painful breasts, restlessness, and tremors.

○   **What position should a female be placed in when performing a pelvic exam?**

The lithotomy position.

○   **What is the *most common* cancer in women?**

Breast cancer.

○　**What is the leading cause of cancer deaths in women?**

Lung cancer.

○　**What is the second leading cause of cancer deaths in women?**

Breast cancer. It affects one of eight women in the USA, and its incidence increases with age. It rarely occurs in men.

○　**Name the risk factors for breast cancer:**

Family history of breast cancer, inherited gene factors (BRCA1 and BRCA2), diabetes, HTN, obesity, lack of breast-feeding, use of estrogen replacement therapy for menopausal symptoms, high-fat diet, history of first pregnancy after age 30, early onset of menarche (before age 12), and late menopause (after age 55).

○　**How much increased lifetime risk for breast cancer is there for women with a known BRCA1 mutation?**

Normal women have an 11% chance of breast cancer; the risk increases to 80% for women with BRCA1 mutation.

○　**As a medsurg nurse you can counsel women on how to perform a breast self-examination. What percentage of breast cancers is discovered by self-examination?**

90%. The breast self-exam (BSE) should be done monthly, at about the same time during the menstrual cycle to allow consistency of exam in case of tenderness or swelling. A mammogram is recommended yearly after age 40.

○　**What is the *most common* treatment for breast cancer?**

Surgery. For some patients who can't undergo surgery or who have inflammatory carcinoma, these patients will need radiation therapy and other measures.

○　**Name the five types of breast surgery that could be performed in the appropriate setting:**

Lumpectomy (tumorectomy), quadrantectomy, simple mastectomy, modified radical mastectomy, and radical mastectomy.

○　**What is the *most common* cancer of the female reproductive system?**

Cervical cancer. It is more common in noncaucasian women, between ages 30 and 50.

○　**What are the risk factors for cervical cancer?**

The number one risk factor is infection with human papilloma virus (HPV) causing 90% of cervical cancer; other risks include multiple male sex partners, long-term use of cigarettes and birth control pills, diet low in vitamin C and carotene, exposure to herpes simplex virus type 2, and first intercourse at a young age.

○　**What are the three categories of treatment for most cancers, including cervical cancer?**

Radiation therapy, surgery, and chemotherapy.

○　**What is endometriosis?**

The endometrial cells that normally line the uterus are somehow displaced into the peritoneum, causing ectopic tissue potentially near or on any organ, including the ovaries, fallopian tubes, cul-de-sac, and other places. These misplaced endometrial cells respond to normal ovarian hormone stimulation, thus during menstruation the ectopic endometrial tissue becomes secretory and bleeds, causing pressure and inflammation of the involved area. It is more common between ages 30 and 40, and causes up to 45% of female infertility. Laparoscopy is usually used to diagnose. Treatment is usually a combination of surgery and medications, but is dependent upon the patient's age, stage of disease, symptoms, and desire to have children.

○ **What is the *most common* fatal gynecologic cancer and the fifth leading cause of cancer death in women?**

Ovarian cancer. It is most common between ages 50 and 60. No early screening tests exist for ovarian cancer, except for CA-125 tumor marker, and possibly transvaginal ultrasound and CT scan.

○ **What is the leading cause of cancer death in men?**

Lung cancer.

○ **What is the second leading cause of cancer death in men?**

Prostate cancer. It is also the most common type of cancer overall, usually adenocarcinoma. Early prostate cancer is asymptomatic. About 50% of patients have advanced stages or have metastasized by the time it's discovered.

○ **What palliative treatments for prostate cancer exist?**

Radiation therapy, suppressive hormone therapy, chemotherapy, cryosurgery, repeated TURP (transurethral resection of the prostate), and measures for pain control.

○ **What are the *most common* infections in the United States?**

STDs, or sexually transmitted diseases. There are more than 21 types of diseases, all of which can be prevented.

○ **What is the *most common* type of cancer in men between ages 15 and 25?**

Testicular cancer. It is more common in younger men.

○ **What percentage of testicular cancer can be "cured" if detected early?**

Up to 95%.

○ **What can medsurg nurses tell men to do that could save their lives?**

Educate men to perform routine testicular self-examination, which improves the likelihood of early detection and intervention. Pain is not a common feature, as less than 20% of patients have any pain early on.

CHAPTER 13 Dermatology Pearls

○ **What type of rash is seen with toxic shock syndrome (TSS)?**

Blanching erythroderma which resolves in 3 days and is followed by a desquamation (full thickness). This typically occurs between the 6th and 14th day with peeling prominent on the hands and feet.

○ **What type of reaction is erythema multiforme (EM)?**

Hypersensitivity.

Bullae are subepidermal, the dermis is edematous, and a lymphatic infiltrate may be present around the capillaries and venules. In children, infections are the most important causes and in adults, drugs and malignancies. EM is often seen during epidemics of adenovirus, atypical pneumonia, and histoplasmosis.

○ **A patient presents with fever, myalgias, malaise, and arthralgias. On exam, findings include bullous lesions of the lips, eyes, and nose. The patient indicates eating is very painful. What syndrome does this describe?**

Stevens-Johnson syndrome has a mortality of 5–10% and may have significant complications including corneal ulceration, panophthalmitis, corneal opacities, anterior uveitis, blindness, hematuria, renal tubular necrosis, and progressive renal failure. Scarring of the foreskin and stenosis of the vagina can occur. Treatment in a burn unit is supportive; steroids may provide symptomatic relief but are not of proven value, and may be contraindicated.

○ **How quickly will people react to the Toxicodendron antigen?**

Contact dermatitis from poison ivy, poison oak, or other toxicodendron plants typically develops within 2 days of exposure; cases have been reported in as quickly as 8 hours to as long as 10 days. Lesions appear in a linear arrangement of papulovesicles or erythema. Fluid from vesicles does not contain antigen and does not transmit the dermatitis.

○ **What medication is given for the treatment of poison ivy?**

Oral steroids such as prednisone, given in large doses for 4–5 days and tapering off over the following few weeks.

○ **What is a furuncle?**

Deep-inflammatory nodule which grows out of superficial folliculitis. Increasingly, the more frequent cause is MRSA (methicillin-resistant Staphylococcus aeureus)

○ **What is a carbuncle?**

Deep abscess that interconnects and extends into the subcutaneous tissue. Commonly seen in patients with diabetes, folliculitis, steroid use, obesity, heavy perspiration, and areas of friction.

○ **What is a pilonidal abscess?**

Abscess which occurs in the gluteal fold as a result of disruption of the epithelial surface. They do not originate from rectal crypts. The bacteria are most commonly from the cutaneous surface.

○ **What is the treatment of a tetanus-prone wound?**

Surgical debridement, 3,000–10,000 units of human tetanus immune globulin [TIG (h), (Hyper-tet)] IM (do not inject into wound), tetanus vaccination updated, penicillin G, or metronidazole if indicated for significantly contaminated wounds.

○ **What is the *most common* cause of gas gangrene?**

Clostridium perfringens (*C. perfringens*). The first symptom is a sensation of weight or heaviness in the muscle followed by severe pain.

○ **What are the *most common* causes of allergic contact dermatitis?**

Poison oak, poison ivy, and poison sumac. They are responsible for more cases of contact dermatitis than all the other allergens combined.

○ **Why does scratching spread poison oak and ivy?**

The antigenic resin contaminates the hands and fingernails, and is thereby spread by rubbing or scratching. A single contaminated finger can produce more than 500 reactive groups of lesions. However, once the skin or hands have been thoroughly washed with soap and water, then scratching does not "spread" the poison ivy. Instead, the body will have an inflammatory allergic reaction of varying places over time, thus giving the appearance that the rash is "spreading."

○ **How is the antigen of poison oak or poison ivy inactivated?**

Careful washing with soap and water removes the oil-like poison ivy/oak antigen. Special attention must be paid to the fingernails, otherwise the antigenic resin can be carried for weeks. Also, the gloves, clothing, and tools that were contaminated with poison ivy oil should be thoroughly cleaned.

○ **Where is the *most common* site of eruption of herpes zoster (shingles)?**

The thorax, usually along one or two dermatomes in distribution. Unlike chicken pox, shingles can recur several times.

○ **Tinea capitis is most commonly seen in what age group?**

Children aged 4–14. This is a fungal infection of the scalp that begins as a papule around one hair shaft and then spreads to other follicles. The infection can cause the hairs to break off, leaving little black dot stumps and patches of alopecia. Trichophyton tonsurans is responsible for 90% of the cases. Wood's lamp examination will fluoresce only Microsporum infections, which are responsible for the remaining 10%. This is also called "ringworm of the scalp." It may be seen in all ages and an outbreak can occur in nursing home patients.

○ **Describe petechia.**

Tiny, round, purplish-red spots that appear on the skin and mucous membranes as a result of intradermal or submucosal hemorrhage.

○ **What is purpura?**

Any purple skin discoloration caused by blood extravasation.

○ **A butterfly rash across the bridge of the nose is a characteristic sign of what connective tissue disorder?**

Systemic lupus erythematosus (SLE).

○ **What are the early indications of gangrene?**

Edema, pain, redness, tissue darkening, and coldness in the affected body part.

○ **What is the *most common* allergic reaction to penicillin?**

Rash.

○ **What is dry gangrene?**

Tissue that is uninfected and mummified with a tendency to self-amputate.

○ **What is wet gangrene?**

Tissue that is moist, infected, swollen, and painful. A rapid spread of infection is noted.

○ **An 18-year-old female admitted for asthma exacerbation is also noted later to be complaining of intense itching in the webs between her fingers that worsens at night. On close examination, you see a few small squiggly lines 1 cm × 1 mm where the patient has been scratching herself. What do you suspect?**

Scabies. Scabies are due to the mite Sarcoptes scabiei var. hominis. Scabies are spread by close contact; therefore, all household contacts should also be treated.

○ **Where are Koplik's spots most commonly found?**

Opposite the lower molars on the buccal mucosa. They can be as small as grains of sand and are commonly grayish-white with red areolae. They occasionally bleed.

○ **Describe the symptoms and signs of varicella (chicken pox).**

The onset of varicella rash is 1–2 days after prodromal symptoms of slight malaise, anorexia, and fever. The rash begins on the trunk and scalp, appearing as faint macules and later becoming vesicles, also known as a pattern called "dew drop on a rose petal."

○ **A 60-year-old patient presents complaining of greasy, red, scaly plaques in her eyebrows, eyelids, and nose that are spreading to the nasolabial folds. What do you suspect?**

The above patient has seborrheic dermatitis. This can occur in anyone but is also a common problem in patients with HIV and Parkinson's disease. The infant form of the disease is "cradle cap."

○   **A 72-year-old female comes to the hospital complaining of a painful red rash with crops of blisters on erythematous bases in a band-like distribution on the right side of her lower back spreading down and out toward her hip. What do you suspect?**

Shingles or herpes zoster disease. This is due to a reactivation of the dormant varicella virus in the sensory root ganglia of a patient with a history of chicken pox. The rash is in the distribution of the dermatome, in this case L5. It is most common in the elderly population or in patients who are immunocompromised. Treatment is with acyclovir and oral analgesics. This will help decrease the postherpetic neuralgia that is frequently associated with the disease.

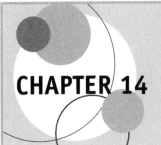

Patient Care Management Pearls

CHAPTER 14

○ **What is one of the most reliable methods of client identification?**

Comparison of client ID bands with the chart information. Never rely solely on the patient as a means of identification. Medications and physical conditions can affect a client's response.

○ **Why is crutch walking often an impractical goal for the elderly patient?**

The strength required for crutch walking and the coordination necessary is often impaired in the elderly. Instead, consider a walker or wheelchair or other device.

○ **A client calls you and states that she has chest pain, feels short of breath, is sweaty, nauseated, and has a history of heart problems. What should you do?**

Tell the patient to hang up and call 911. There is no way to tell for sure, but the patient is describing symptoms of a heart attack which could be life threatening.

○ **What is required prior to an invasive procedure?**

Informed consent.

○ **What is the purpose of the Z-track intramuscular injection technique?**

To seal medication deep into the muscle, thereby minimizing skin irritation and staining.

○ **What are the five stages of the nursing process?**

Assessment
Nursing diagnosis
Planning
Implementation
Evaluation

○ **What does the acronym SOAP represent?**

It represents a format used to write nursing progress notes. The S stands for subjective data, O for objective data, A for assessment, and P for plan.

○   **In the SOAP format, who provides the subjective data?**

The patient.

○   **What are the three names given to all pharmaceutical drugs?**

The generic name, which is used in official publications.
    The trade or brand name, which is selected by the pharmaceutical company.
    The chemical name that describes the chemical composition of the drug.

○   **What gauge needle should be used for subcutaneous injections?**

25 gauge needle.

○   **Where should you secure the loose end of a restraint after first attaching it to a bed-ridden patient?**

The bed frame or springs.

○   **What is a living will?**

A witnessed document that states a patient's desire for certain types of care and treatment.

○   **What are the five rights of medication administration?**

The right route, the right time, the right dose, the right medication, and the right patient.

○   **Before administering any medication to a client, what should you check?**

Drug allergies.

○   **When can medication be forced upon a client?**

Only if the patient poses a threat to himself or others without it.

○   **What metabolic abnormality can occur as a result of multiple blood transfusions?**

Hypocalcemia can occur due to the presence of the preservative EDTA, which binds calcium.

○   **Why should topical nitroglycerin be removed from the chest before defibrillation?**

Topical medications can cause electrical arcing.

○   **T/F: Unwitnessed cardiac arrests will require an autopsy to be performed by the medical examiner.**

False. Forensic examination is done when the cause of death is suspected of being unnatural, while a cardiac arrest is considered natural. However, most states require notification of the coroner even though an autopsy will likely not be done.

○   **Which medication is used to counteract soft tissue necrosis after extravasation of dopamine hydrochloride (Intropin)?**

Phentolamine (Regitine).

○   **What is the *most common* initial emotional change resulting from critical incident stress?**

Panic

○ **What is the primary nursing diagnosis for the kidney transplant patient not following treatment protocols?**

Ineffective management of therapeutic regimen.

○ **What is the primary nursing diagnosis in a patient with a kidney transplant?**

Increased risk for infection.

○ **When talking with a non-English speaking individual, which word should be avoided?**

Not. This word can be lost in a sentence and create the opposite meaning.

○ **What is the priority nursing diagnosis for a patient who presents with peritonitis?**

Decreased intravascular fluid volume.

○ **What nursing intervention is appropriate for the sudden-cardiac-death survivor?**

Notifying the patient's support system, including family, friends, and clergy.

○ **What is the primary nursing diagnosis for a patient with acute congestive heart failure?**

Decreased cardiac output.

○ **Why should the Allen test be performed before inserting an arterial line?**

To ensure that collateral circulation in the hand is adequate.

○ **What is the priority nursing diagnosis for a patient with an open, depressed skull fracture?**

Risk for infection related to trauma.

○ **What is the priority nursing diagnosis for a patient with endocarditis?**

Altered cardiopulmonary tissue perfusion.

○ **What nursing diagnosis is of concern for a patient with a mandibular fracture?**

Ineffective airway clearance.

○ **What is the most accurate nursing diagnosis for a patient who was sexually assaulted?**

Rape-trauma syndrome. This refers to both the acute and the long-term phases experienced by the victim of a sexual assault.

○ **What is the primary nursing diagnosis for a patient with myasthenia gravis?**

Ineffective breathing pattern related to weakness of respiratory muscles.

○ **What is the primary nursing diagnosis for a patient who sustained an eyelid laceration?**

Risk for infection related to a break in skin integrity.

○ **What is the most important diagnosis in a patient with a pulmonary contusion?**

Impaired gas exchange related to blood extravasation.

○ **A patient presents to the hospital admission area after spilling organophosphates on himself. Before assessing the patient, what should the nurse do?**

Protect themselves, protect their coworkers and patients in the hospital or clinic, and before initiating patient care, have the patient leave or be removed from the building. Off-gassing and contamination inside are dangerous. Appropriate PPE should be done first and then decontamination and stabilizing treatment can be done, and when clean, the patient can be brought back inside the hospital or clinic.

○ **What is the priority nursing diagnosis for an ethanol intoxicated, semiresponsive patient?**

Ineffective airway clearance related to alcohol intoxication.

○ **What is the primary nursing diagnosis for a patient with pyelonephritis?**

Risk for fluid volume deficit.

○ **What is the primary nursing diagnosis for an acutely burned patient?**

Fluid volume deficit.

○ **What is the best nursing diagnosis to explain the effect of cyanide poisoning?**

Impaired gas exchange.

○ **What is the primary nursing diagnosis for a patient with an intestinal obstruction?**

Fluid volume deficit.

○ **What is the primary nursing diagnosis for a patient with eclampsia?**

Risk of injury, seizures, death, poor infant outcome possible.

○ **What is the primary nursing diagnosis for a patient with angina?**

Altered cardiopulmonary tissue perfusion.

○ **What is the primary nursing diagnosis for a patient with an esophageal rupture?**

Risk for infection.

○ **A trauma patient receives a large amount of room temperature crystalloids and refrigerated blood. What nursing diagnosis best describes the potential effect?**

Hypothermia.

○ **What is a bruit?**

A vascular sound that resembles a heart murmur. It results from turbulent flow through a diseased or partially obstructed artery.

○ **Where on the body does jaundice first manifest?**

The sclera.

○ **How long should you count an irregular pulse?**

60 seconds.

○ **What is the bell of the stethoscope used for?**

To hear low-pitched sounds such as heart murmurs.

○ **What is the purpose of the diaphragm of the stethoscope?**

It is used to hear high-pitched sounds such as breath sounds.

○ **How much of the arm should a blood pressure cuff cover?**

1/3 of the patient's upper arm.

○ **How far should the blood pressure cuff be from the antecubital fossa?**

One inch.

○ **Following a lumbar puncture what nursing care should be provided?**

Provide emotional support, apply a bandage to the site and hold pressure for a short period. Keep patient flat for 6 hours.

○ **What is considered a normal central venous pressure?**

2–3 mm Hg (or 3–15 cm of water).

○ **Why is CVP monitored?**

To assess the need for fluid replacement, estimate blood volume deficits, and evaluate circulatory pressure in the right atrium.

○ **What patient position will enhance the murmur of mitral stenosis?**

Left lateral decubitus.

○ **What is optimal patient position and maneuver for auscultation of aortic insufficiency?**

Have the patient sit up and lean forward with the hands tightly clasped. During exhalation, listen at the left sternal border.

○ **What antihypertensive agent may induce cyanide poisoning?**

Nitroprusside. One molecule of sodium nitroprusside contains 5 molecules of cyanide. In order to prevent toxicity, sodium thiosulfate should be infused with sodium nitroprusside at a ratio of 10:1, thiosulfate to nitroprusside.

○ **Following the administration of morphine sulfate, what important adverse reactions should you watch for?**

Low blood pressure and decreased respirations.

○ **The physician orders a nitroglycerin drip, and so you obtain an IV infusion pump for administration. What is the rationale for this?**

The infusion pump will ensure that the medication is titrated accurately.

CHAPTER 15

Organization and Personnel Management Pearls

○ **A nurse's aide refuses to go into an HIV positive client's room because she is afraid of contracting AIDS. How should you respond?**

Teach the aide how the HIV is transmitted and the concept of universal precautions. Education and reassurance should solve the major issue. Let the employee know what your expectations are and what normal nursing protocols include.

○ **A client is being admitted for bacterial meningitis. What type of room would be the most appropriate?**

A private room to reduce the spread of the infection. If the meningitis is caused by a contagious pathogen, then additional precautions and prophylactic treatment may be indicated for close contacts and family members.

○ **When delegating responsibilities to other team members, what two factors are considered the most important?**

The appropriateness and the fairness of the assignment.

○ **If a member of the nursing team appears to be under the influence of drugs or alcohol, what action should you take?**

Notify your immediate supervisor and remove the nurse from her assignment.

○ **What is quality assurance?**

A method of determining whether nursing actions and practices meet established standards.

○ **A 30-year-old intoxicated male is brought to the medsurg floor. On transfer to a treatment stretcher, he becomes violent and verbally abusive. What is the first priority of the medsurg nurse?**

Protect themselves, the fellow staff and existing patients, and the abusive patient/family from physical harm.

○ **This same patient refuses medical care and wishes to leave. What is the appropriate action?**

If the patient is intoxicated and acting irrationally, then that patient should be detained until a full medical evaluation can be performed. If the patient is not intoxicated, irrational, or exhibiting signs of altered mental status, then the patient may be allowed to sign out against medical advice (AMA). However, all reasonable efforts should be expended to try to get the patient to complete medical evaluation and treatment appropriately.

○   **What qualifications should be met before a patient can leave against medical advice (AMA)?**

The patient must be mentally competent to understand the consequences of refusing care, and must not be hypoxic, hypoglycemic, psychotic, under the influence of mind-altering drugs, or have a history of recent head injury.

○   **It is determined that this patient is competent to refuse care. What should then be done?**

Consequences of refusal should be explained in detail and documented on the patient's chart. The patient should sign an AMA form and be told they are welcome to return for further care. Ideally there should be several witnesses. The patient's physician should be involved if at all possible, and must be told as soon as possible of the crisis and refusal of care. Often times once the patient's concerns or misunderstandings are addressed, then the patient is more calm, cooperative, and less likely to refuse medical care.

○   **A medsurg nurse is being criticized for taking too long to see and process patients upon arrival to the floor. Which continuous quality improvement (CQI) tool might be used to assist the staff and manager in identifying the real cause of the delay?**

A flowchart. This is a pictorial representation of the steps of the process, which helps to delineate the process so that it can be improved.

○   **A 17-year-old female with flulike symptoms is admitted to the floor by her 19-year-old sister. Permission to treat should be received from whom?**

The patient's parent, guardian, or appropriate adult with signed permission from the parent(s).

○   **What is the process of critical incident stress debriefing (CISD) used for?**

CISD offers immediate debriefing to individuals after a critically emotional or traumatic situation. This is typically assisted by uninvolved, objective persons who are trained in this area. CISD assists in dealing with immediate emotional reactions by allowing staff members to talk about their feelings, and to discuss positive ways to deal with the emotions felt by medical staff members.

○   **What is the nurse's first priority in research?**

Rights of the human subjects.

○   **How should a nurse prepare for, and answer questions during a deposition or court trial?**

The nurse should legally obtain and beforehand review the chart and all related materials and answer all questions honestly, keeping terminology simple and direct. Answer only the questions asked, briefly and without excessive language, while offering no information not directly sought.

○   **How should clothes be removed and processed from a victim who sustained a gunshot wound?**

Preserve the evidence as best possible. Cut around any knife or bullet holes in clothing. All clothing should be labeled as to their source, the patient's name, age, date, and time collected, and placed in a paper bag (not plastic bag) to preserve evidence. The chain of evidence should be documented and maintained in proper fashion, and given to the involved law enforcement officers appropriately.

○   **When does the receiving hospital's liability begin, related to patient transport?**

Liability begins once the receiving hospital accepts the patient.

○ **What physical abnormality is most commonly reported from critical incident stress?**

Sleep disturbance.

○ **What is the best way to increase acceptance when introducing changes to a nursing unit?**

Always explain the reason for all changes made. If possible, get input from the involved nurses during formulation of the new policy or change, and make appropriate modifications to the changes prior to actual incorporation.

○ **What type of budget covers supplies, unit equipment, repairs, and overhead?**

Operational budget.

○ **What type of budget covers land, buildings, and expensive durable equipment?**

Capital budget.

○ **What is the purpose of research in nursing?**

Generate a scientific knowledge base for validating and improving nursing practice.

CHAPTER 16

Legal Issues and Quality Improvement Pearls

○ **What is quality improvement?**

A method of determining whether nursing actions and practices meet established standards.

○ **What problem-solving method generates as many solutions as possible?**

Brainstorming.

○ **For negligence to be proven in court, what four elements must be present?**

(1) Duty (accepting responsibility for care), (2) breach of duty (not providing care according to accepted standards), (3) damage (damage must have occured), and (4) proximate cause (a cause-and-effect relationship between the damage and the breach of duty must exist).

○ **What is a fishbone (cause–effect) diagram?**

A CQI tool used to help generate ideas and organize theories about possible causes of the observed problem.

○ **What are the components of informed consent?**

Providing a description of the procedure, a discussion of any alternatives treatments, and a discussion of the risks and benefits of the procedure.

○ **At which point is the patient owed a duty of care?**

Upon arrival to the hospital, emergency department, or nursing unit.

○ **How should documentation errors in the medical record be corrected?**

Draw a single line through the error, date and initial it and state the reason for the correction.

○ **Which document outlines a patient's wishes regarding emergency treatment if the patient is unable to speak due to a disability?**

Advanced directive.

○ **What is a durable power of attorney?**

A legal document that gives another person the power to make health care decisions for the patient if the patient is unable to make own decisions.

○ **What code compels a nurse to treat a homeless patient with multiple minor complaints with dignity?**

Code of Ethics for Nurses.

○ **What is the definition of a tort?**

A civil wrong committed against a person or property that can be remedied with money paid to the plaintiff.

○ **What is breach of duty?**

A failure to meet the accepted standards of care for a patient.

○ **When does the patient and nurse confidentiality not apply?**

Protective privilege ends where the public peril begins. It is the duty of the nurse or physician to alert proper authorities and the threatened individual when a patient (or family member) threatens another person with bodily injury or harm.

○ **A medsurg nurse takes further history from a recently admitted 16-year-old patient with fever and UTI. Subsequent history suggests that this patient has been sexually abused. However, the mother does not want to tell the police because the assailant is her boyfriend. What should you do?**

The nurse must report the crime to the authorities because he/she has a duty of care to the patient who has been harmed. The physician should be involved, and appropriate contact to law enforcement and child protective services should be made. The child must not be allowed to leave until the situation has been investigated and safety of the child determined.

○ **What information should be recorded on every woman of child-bearing age who presents to the emergency department or other hospital unit?**

Date of last menstrual period.

○ **What is the best method for protecting yourself against possible negligence or malpractice litigation?**

Provide and document care within accepted standards.

○ **What is the *most common* unintentional tort involving health care personnel?**

Negligence.

○ **What does the Consolidated Omnibus Budget Reconciliation Act of 1989 (COBRA) require a hospital to do if they can't provide a required service for a patient?**

Medically screen and stabilize the patient before transporting to an appropriate facility.

○ **If you suspect child abuse, but you are not sure, should it be reported?**

Yes. It is your legal obligation.

○ **When suspecting child abuse, what are some important assessments that should be documented on the patient's chart?**

The behavior of the patient and any physical findings. The exact words used by the victim and related contacts should be documented in writing. These will be important if the case goes to court.

○ **A fellow nurse states that she suspects child abuse with one of her clients, but fears reporting it because the patient's father is a lawyer. How should you respond to this nurse?**

A health care professional cannot be sued for reporting a suspected child abuse case. Proceed with contacting authorities per protocol and legal obligation.

○ **What are the typical criteria for brain death (these may vary from state to state)?**

Unresponsiveness to painful stimuli, absence of spontaneous respiration or muscle movement, and loss of brainstem function (as evidenced by fixed, dilated pupils, and absence of reflexes, and a flat electroencephalogram).

○ **What is the standard of care for victims of domestic violence currently recommended by JCAHO, the AMA, and the CDC?**

  (1) Establish a confidential system to identify domestic violence victims.

  (2) Document the abuse.

  (3) Collect physical evidence.

  (4) Evaluate safety issues and potential for lethality or suicide.

  (5) Formulate a safety plan with the victim.

  (6) Advise the victim of all his/her options and resources.

  (7) Refer for counseling and other services, including legal assistance.

  (8) Coordinate with law enforcement.

  (9) Transport to a shelter if desired or needed.

(10) Follow-up with a domestic violence advocate.

CHAPTER 17 Wound Care Pearls

○ **What is the initial intervention for a patient with external bleeding?**

Direct pressure.

○ **Traumatic wounds account for what percent of hospital visits?**

10%.

○ **How quickly do wounds recover their tensile strength?**

50% at 40 days; 90% at 150 days.

○ **A patient has a wood splinter in the finger. The doctor is busy. Should you go ahead and have the patient soak the finger while waiting?**

No, wounds that involve wood should not be soaked in liquid as the wood might disintegrate and make it very difficult to remove. Also, recent studies have proven that "soaking the wound" actually increases the risk for wound infection. Instead, an initial simple gross decontamination followed by timely physician exam, irrigation, and wound repair are noted ways to decrease wound infections.

○ **What are the stages of wound healing?**

Hemostasis
Inflammation
Epithelialization
Angiogenesis
Fibroplasia
Wound contracture
Scar remolding

○ **What is the *most common* foreign body?**

Soil. Clay-contaminated soils and soils with organic material have high potential infection

○ **What types of wounds usually require consultation?**

Wounds that involve

significant loss of epidermis.
tendons, nerves, or vessels.

face that requires extensive reconstruction.

amputation.

loss of function.

open fracture or joint space.

tarsal plate of the eyelid or lacrimal duct.

multiple trauma.

○ **When should epinephrine be avoided in wound closure?**

Fingers, toes, nose, and penis.

○ **T/F: Hair should be clipped and not shaved.**

True, shaving can increase infection.

○ **T/F: High-pressure irrigation increases the risk of infection.**

False, it will decrease bacterial counts, remove foreign bodies, and decrease infections.

○ **T/F: Wound scrubbing or soaking is not effective in cleaning contaminated wounds.**

True.

○ **A pneumatic tourniquet can be inflated on an extremity to more than a patient's systolic blood pressure for how long?**

2 hours without damage to underlying vessels or nerves.

○ **What are the 4 Cs in determining muscle viability?**

Color, consistency, contraction, and circulation

○ **For how long can wound care be delayed before proliferation of bacteria that may result in infection?**

3 hours.

○ **What mechanisms of injury create wounds that are most susceptible to infection?**

Compression or tension injuries. They are 100 times more susceptible to infection.

○ **What types of wounds result in the majority of tetanus cases?**

Lacerations, punctures, and crush injuries.

○ **Characterize tetanus prone wounds.**

Age of wound: >6 hours.

Configuration: stellate wound.

Depth: >1 cm.

Mechanism of injury: missile, crush, burn, frostbite.

Signs of infection: present.

Devitalized tissue: present.

Contaminants: present.

Denervated and/or ischemic tissue: present.

○ **How long does it take for a watertight seal to form in surgical incisions?**

About 24 hours.

○ **When does the maturation phase of a normally healing wound occur?**

About 3 weeks after injury.

○ **T/F: Healed wounds are as strong as unwounded tissue.**

False.

○ **What is the *most common* cause of wound healing deficiency?**

Lack of vitamin C.

○ **What has been proven to decrease the pain of local anesthetic administration?**

Buffering the lidocaine with sodium bicarbonate (1 part bicarb to 9 parts lidocaine) (do not use bicarbonate with mepivicaine or bupivicaine).

Decreasing the speed of injection.

Use of a subdermal injection instead of superficial or intradermal injections.

Topical coolant spray on the skin prior to needle insertion.

○ **Why is epinephrine added to local anesthesia?**

To increase the duration of the anesthesia.

Epinephrine also causes vasoconstriction and decreased bleeding, which weakens tissue defenses and may potentially increase the incidence of wound infection.

○ **What local anesthetic, ester or amide, is responsible for most allergic reactions?**

Esters such as procaine.

○ **What is the dose of bacteria necessary to cause wound infection without a foreign body and with a foreign body?**

Without foreign body—$>10^6$ bacteria/gm of tissue.

With foreign body—100 bacteria.

○ **Bacterial endocarditis secondary to soft tissue infections may be caused by which two organisms?**

Staphylococcus aureus and *Staphylococcus epidermidis*.

○ **What factors increase the likelihood of wound infection?**

Dirty or contaminated wounds, stellate or crushing wounds, wounds longer than 5 cm, wounds older than 6 hours, and infection prone anatomic sites.

○ **What are the three categories of wound closure?**

Primary—healing with suture, staples, adhesives.
Secondary—healing by granulation.
Tertiary—delayed primary closure.

○ **What factors determine the ultimate appearance of a scar?**

Static and dynamic skin tension on surrounding skin, family genetics, and history of keloid formation in the patient after past injuries.

○ **Which has lower resistance to infection, sutures or staples?**

Sutures are at slightly higher risk of infection compared to staples.

○ **How long should one wait before delayed primary closure?**

4 days. This will decrease the infection rate and is used for severely contaminated wounds.

○ **How long do sutures maintain their tensile strength?**

Nonabsorbable—more than 60 days.
Absorbable—less than 60 days.

○ **When should silk sutures be avoided?**

In contaminated wounds as they potentiate infection and bacteria can spread via the fibers.

○ **T/F: Anyone with facial trauma should be questioned about the possibility of domestic violence.**

True.

○ **T/F: Eyebrows should never be clipped or shaved.**

True, they are valuable landmarks and may not regrow.

○ **Which eyelid wounds should be referred to an ophthalmologist?**

Inner surface of the lid
Lid margins
Lacrimal duct involvement
Presence of ptosis
Extension into tarsal plate

○ **Following a nasal injury, what should be ruled out?**

The septum should be inspected for a hematoma.
Bluish swelling in the septum confirms a hematoma which needs to be evacuated.
Bilateral hematomas should be drained by a specialist.

○ **What region of the hand is innervated by the ulnar nerve, radial nerve, and median nerve?**

Unlar—5th and half of 4th

Radial—posterior of hand, posterior half of 2nd, 3rd, 4th, and 5th fingers.

Median—anterior hand, 1st, 2nd, 3rd, and half of 4th finger.

○ **How do you test motor function of the radial, ulnar, and median nerves?**

Radial—wrist and digit extension.

Ulnar—Finger abduction and adduction, thumb adduction.

Median—Thumb flexion, opposition, and abduction.

○ **A patient arrives to the medsurg floor with a complaint of inability to hitchhike, as ever since a knife fight he has been unable to extend his thumb. What nerve has been damaged?**

Radial nerve.

○ **T/F: Lacerations to the extensor tendons over the distal IP joint cause a mallet deformity.**

True.

○ **T/F: Lacerations over the proximal IP joint cause a boutonniere deformity.**

True.

○ **How do you check the integrity of the Achilles tendon?**

Thompson Test—belly of the gastrocnemius is squeezed while the patient kneels on a chair. An intact Achilles tendon produces plantar flexion of the foot.

○ **What percent of foot lacerations become infected?**

18–34%, therefore consider antibiotic prophylaxis.

○ **A wound which occurred while wading in fresh water often gets what type of infection?**

Aeromonas.

Rx—Fluoroquinolone in adults, trimethoprim-sulfamethoxazole in children.

○ **What is the *most common* organism found in a puncture wound?**

Staph aureus.

Rx—dicloxacillin or Fluoroquinolone.

○ **Gabriella Sabatini, the famous tennis star, presents to your "fast-track" after stepping on a nail that went right through her favorite, oldest pair of tennis shoes. What organism might infect her puncture wound?**

Pseudomonas aeruginosa.

Osteomyelitis may occur if it involves the bone.

Plantar wounds, especially those through tennis shoes, should receive prophylactic antibiotics.

Fluoroquinolone in adults, cephalexin in children.

○ **What is the common bacteria seen in cat bite wounds which can also occur with dog bites?**

Pasteurella multocida.

○   **A patient presents with a human bite wound that was inflicted while he was in a mental ward. What bacterium is likely?**

Eikenella corrodens, anerobic streptococci, and Staphylococcus.

○   **What percentage of dog and cat bites become infected?**

About 10% of dog and 50% of cat bites become infected.

Pasteurella multocida infects 30% of dog and 50% of cat bites.

○   **If a dog bite becomes infected within 24 hours, what is the most likely bacterium?**

P. multocida.

Rx—penicillin, ciprofloxsin, and trimethoprim/sulfamethoxazole.

If after 24 hours, Strep or Staph are usually the cause.

Rx—dicloxacillin or cephalosporin.

○   **A 16-year-old presents with headache, fever, malaise, and tender regional lymphadenopathy about a week after a cat bite. A tender papule develops at the site. Diagnosis?**

Cat-scratch disease. Usually develops 3 days to 6 weeks following a cat bite or scratch.

The papule typically blisters and heals with eschar formation or a transient macular or vesicular rash may develop.

○   **Given the choice, would you rather receive a superficial bite from Fluffy or Rover?**

Rover. Fluffy the cat, has an 80% chance of causing a P. multocida infection.

A cat bite can also cause Cat Scratch disease, 2% of which may develop extension into the CNS, liver, spleen, bone, or skin. Penicillin is the antibiotic of choice.

○   **What is the cause of Cat Scratch disease?**

Bartonella henselae is thought to be the causative organism.

○   **Given the choice, would you rather be bitten by Fluffy or Biff the Bully?**

Fluffy the cat.

Human bites have the highest rate of causing infection.

○   **A patient presents with a small curvilinear laceration over the fourth knuckle on his dominant hand. He reports cutting this on the engine block of his car. How should this wound be considered?**

Treat the wound as if it were a human bite-type wound as this patient may have struck another person in the mouth resulting in a "bite" or cut from the teeth of another person. Patients may not tell the truth if they feel that the police may be called due to suspected altercation/fight. Human bite wounds over the knuckle generally should not be sutured.

Careful exploration for tendon or joint space involvement, along with thorough cleansing, is necessary. Because of the potentially devastating infectious sequelae, antibiotics, and early follow-up care are routine.

○   **T/F: Appropriate prophylaxis for hepatitis B in an unimmunized health care worker who is exposed to hepatitis B infected blood exists.**

True, one of the following treatment options can be performed:

(1) Two doses of hepatitis B immune globulin—one immediately and 1 month later or

(2) a single dose of immune globulin and initiation of hepatitis B vaccine series.

○ **T/F: Aerosol exposures place a health care worker at the greatest risk to seroconvert from a blood-borne pathogen.**

False, the greatest risk is from a penetrating sharps injury in which the sharp was a hollow needle that was used in an infected blood source. The risk is particularly increased in cases where a hollow-bore needle is involved, the wound is deeply penetrating, and/or blood is injected.

○ **T/F: The seroconversion rate for a health care worker exposed from a sharps injury to HIV-infected blood is approximately 1.5%.**

False, the seroconversion rate for a health care worker exposed from a sharps injury to HIV-infected blood is approximately 0.3%.

○ **T/F: The seroconversion rate from exposure to blood from a HIV-infected source patient can be decreased by 67% if PEP (postexposure prophylaxis) medications are started within 2–3 hours after exposure.**

True. The health care worker, police officer, or other person who is exposed to blood or other body fluids from an AIDS or HIV-positive patient should be rapidly seen and counseled, and if the injury and risks are significant, then the 3-medicine PEP kit should be taken initially within 2–3 hours, followed by daily medications for 1 month followed by re-evaluation. The GI side effects are considerable and many people will stop the medications due to side effects or after the source patient has been shown (if possible or known) to be HIV –negative.

○ **T/F: Baseline laboratory studies are indicated for a health care worker who sustains a needlestick injury from a patient source.**

True, baseline laboratory studies include testing for antibodies to HIV and hepatitis B and C panels.

○ **What are the key prophylactic antibiotics to remember?**

Intraoral laceration—penicillin.

Human bites—amoxicillin/clavulanate (Augmentin).

Dog bites—amoxicillin/clavulanate.

Cat bites—amoxicillin/clavulanate.

Rubber shoe punctures—ciprofloxacin in adults and cephalexin in children.

○ **When should sutures be removed?**

Face—4–5 days.

Scalp—10 days.

Trunk—10–12 days.

Arm—10–12 days.

Leg—10–12 days.

Hand—10–14 days.

Joint—10–14 days.

Foot—14 days.

If the patient is immunocompromised, on steroids, or elderly then additional days should be added to these times due to impaired wound healing.

CHAPTER 18 Perioperative Pearls

○ **What is the purpose of preoperative clearance?**

To provide a safety checklist, help ensure that the patient is stable and cardiovascularly healthy enough to undergo surgery, and to evaluate for surgical complications.

○ **What are the components of preoperative phase?**

Review of history—paying close attention to recent chest pain, dyspnea, recent illnesses including any fever or cough.

Discuss psychosocial needs, anxiety, fears, family members that will be waiting on patient, etc.

Medications including nonprescription, herbal medications/supplements.

Allergies and sensitivities including any tape, latex, or other products.

Anesthesia history—inquire about previous reactions.

Social history including smoking, alcohol, recreational drugs.

Pain assessment.

Physical assessment including respiratory, cardiac, hepatic, renal, and neurological status.

Preadmission labs, chest x-ray, and EKG for patients over 40.

Preoperative teaching including discussion of NPO status, medications prior to surgery, pre surgical preps, verification of surgical site, prosthetic devices, i.e., glasses, contact lenses, hearing aids, and dentures etc.

○ **Why are patients kept NPO or nothing by mouth after midnight prior to surgery?**

This long held policy is to decrease the risk of aspiration/regurgitation during surgery/anesthesia.

○ **What is the purpose of a preoperative chest x-ray?**

By traditional standards, a chest x-ray is done preoperatively to use for comparison or for postoperatively changes. About 1% of routine chest x-rays show changes or disease and less than 0.1% result in changes in surgical management.

○ **What are typical preoperative laboratory tests?**

A CBC or complete blood count assesses for anemia, specifically a hemoglobin and hematocrit. Basic metabolic profile to include a glucose to screen for diabetes, especially in the elderly populations, a blood urea nitrogen (BUN) to assess renal function and electrolytes. Some surgeons will screen for bleeding disorders with a prothrombin time (PT), and activated partial thromboplastin time (aPTT). Other preexisting conditions may require further testing, i.e., patients taking theophylline, digoxin, Dilantin, Tegretol, lithium, or antiarrhythmics may need medication levels. Urinalysis may be a requirement of some surgeons, especially if urological instrumentation is utilized.

○ **What are some problems that might preclude surgery?**

Infection.

Hemoglobin less than 10 g/dL.

Platelet counts less than 50,000/mm3 (platelets may be corrected with platelet transfusion to increase this level).

Severe malnutrition or bowel sterilization may result in vitamin K deficiency, a decrease in clotting factors resulting in bleeding.

Electrolyte abnormalities. Correction is critical prior to surgery to prevent arrhythmias.

Glucose greater than 200 mg/dL.

Uncontrolled hypertension, some say, no more than 110 diastolic.

Hyperthyroid state, patients should be euthyroid prior to surgery.

○ **What is the American Surgical Association (ASA) physical status classification system?**

It is an assignment of surgical risk as follows:

- Status I: healthy patient.
- Status II: a patient with mild to moderate disease such as anemia, morbid obesity.
- Status III: patients with severe systemic disease that may limit activity such as healed MIs, DM with vascular complications.
- Status IV: patients with incapacitating systemic disease that is life-threatening such as advanced hepatic or renal disease.
- Status V: patients that are not expected to survive such as major trauma, massive PE (pulmonary embolus).

○ **Why is aspirin held prior to surgery?**

Aspirin may inactive platelet function for as long as 10 days after ingestion and therefore may increase bleeding. Nonsteroidal anti-inflammatory drugs (NSAIDs), steroids, and phenothiazines may interfere with platelet function.

○ **What factors increase cardiac risk/complications during surgery?**

MI within the last 6 months.

Third heart sound, S3 or jugular venous distension (JVD).

More than five premature ventricular contractions per minute noted anytime prior to entering the OR.

Poor medical condition such as increased BUN, bedridden patients.

Intrathoracic, Intrapertoneal or aortic surgery.

Emergency surgery.

○ **How long does it take for a watertight seal to form in surgical incisions?**

About 24 hours.

○ **T/F: Healed wounds are as strong as unwounded tissue.**

False.

○ **What are some important preventive measures to avoid bacterial wound contamination?**

Preoperative showers using antimicrobial soaps, i.e., chlorhexidine or providone iodine.

Removal of hair with clippers as shaving promotes infection.

Proper technique during surgery (hand and arm washing, sterile procedures, wound irrigation, pre-op antibiotics, proper surgical technique).

○ **What are the responsibilities of the operating room nurse?**

Confirm patient name and compare to ID band, surgery and site, review informed consent form.

Review chart for history, physical, diagnostic test results, note allergies, and reactions to anesthesia.

Confirm that wigs, prosthetic devices, dentures, jewelry, body piercings etc. have been removed.

Provide emotional support while patient is conscious.

Maintain patient safety and security.

Confirm sponge, needle, and instrument counts are correct.

○ **What are the categories of anesthesia?**

General: body relaxation, decreased sensation, and unconsciousness.

Regional: provides anesthesia of a specific body area without loss of consciousness and given by IV, spinal, or epidural.

Local: provides anesthesia over a limited area given topically or via infiltration.

○ **What are the *most common* antibacterial skin prep scrubs?**

Iodophors, i.e., Betadine.

○ **What are other surgical preparations on the part of the surgical team to reduce infection rates?**

Hand scrubbing for at least 3–5 minutes with an antiseptic prior to each surgical case with either an iodophor or chlorhexidine combined with a detergent.

Face mask to cover the nose and mouth.

Gloves protect both the patient and the surgeon from contamination.

Sterile gowns, booties, and hair covers.

Sterile drapes.

Sterilized instruments.

○ **What are the types of general anesthesia?**

IV medications

    ultra short acting barbiturates, i.e., thiopental, thiamylal, methohexital

    ketamine

    benzodiazepines i.e. diazepam, midazolam

    propofol

    narcotics, i.e., morphine, meperidine, Fentanyl, sufentanil, alfentanil

Inhalation agents such as nitrous oxide, halothane, enflurane, and isoflurane.

Or a combination of the two agents plus muscle relaxers, i.e., succinylcholine, vercuronium, and pancuronium.

○ **What is involved in regional anesthesia?**

Involves blockade of nerve impulses in selected areas of the body usually using local anesthetics, i.e., lidocaine, procaine, tetracaine, etc.

Can be major conduction blockage, i.e., spinal and epidural anesthesia.

Can be peripheral nerve blockage, i.e., plexus vs. individual nerves.

○ **What are the current parameters of monitoring the anesthetized patient?**

Physiologic monitoring to include patient's color, pulse, EKG monitoring, electronic BP and pulse oximetry, temperature by probe, esophageal stethoscope, end CO_2 detection devices, serial ABG devices, nerve stimulation devices, and renal function via Foley catheter.

Despite modern technology, it should not be forgotten that the old standards of monitoring respiratory and heart rate, pupillary reflexes, and "taking good care of the patient" are still necessary.

○ **What types of medical emergencies can occur during surgery that may not be seen immediately or until recovery?**

Stroke

MI

Pulmonary embolus

Reaction to anesthesia

Renal failure/renal damage from anesthetics or intraoperative insults

○ **Is fever usually the result of poor surgical technique?**

In the first 24 hours about 80% of the time, the source of the fever is not found and abates without intervention.

However, pulmonary atelectasis (not fully expanding the lungs) can cause fever and may be corrected by incentive spirometry and increased ambulation.

○ **What are the *most common* causes of fever post-op?**

5 Ws:

wind = atelectasis due to decreased respiratory physiology, more common in the elderly, smokers/COPD pt, obese and upper abdominal surgery. Seen within the first 48 hours and treatment is to perform incentive spirometry, pulmonary physiotherapy and encourage coughing and deep breaths. Chest x-ray to determine pneumonia etc.

wound = check for infection, treat with drainage, antibiotics (usually seen after 5 days).

water = UTI, check urine especially if catheterized.

wonder drugs = drug reactions, although not common.

walking veins = check for DVT, phlebitis from IVs.

○ **T/F: The most common source of infection is from the patient.**

True. Organisms recovered from infections usually come from the patient with the operating team as a secondary source.

○ **What are the other factors that influence wound infections?**

Age

Obesity

Diabetes

Cirrhosis

Uremia

Connective tissue disorders

○ **T/F: Necrotizing wound infection is a common postsurgical complication.**

False, although uncommon, symptoms include crepitus, pain with edematous discoloration, and treatment with surgical debridement and broad spectrum antibiotics.

○ **What are the common causes of postoperative dyspnea?**

Atelectasis (most common). However, pulmonary atelectasis (not fully expanding the lungs) can cause fever and may be corrected by incentive spirometry and increased ambulation.

Aspiration including GERD, food in the stomach, intestinal obstruction, and patients undergoing rapid sequence intubation in emergent situations.

Pneumonia atelectasis, aspiration, and copious secretions are predisposing factors. Usually fever, tachycardia present. Often gram negative or polymicrobial.

Heart failure due to fluid overload (common) especially in patients that have cardiac compromise (MI, dysrhythmias etc.).

Pulmonary embolus is a common post op complication that can result in high morbity and mortality especially if unrecognized.

○ **T/F: Pulmonary embolism is the greatest postsurgical risk.**

True, PE is the leading cause of death of hospitalized patients.

Rate of venous thromboembolism ranges from 7 to 29% for gyn and about 45% in patients with malignant diseases.

Prevalence of DVT after surgery depends on underlying health of the patient and other risk factors.

Those developing PE, die within the first 30 minutes of the event.

PE can occur without clinical evidence in *50–80%* of cases and fatal in *10–20%*.

○ **Classify low, moderate and severe risk of DVT in surgical patients:**

Low (less than 3%): age less than 40 with surgery less than 30 minutes.

Moderate (10–40% risk): age greater than 40 with surgery of any duration without other risk factors.

Severe (40–70% risk): age greater than 40 with the following risk factors:

Prior DVT or PE

Varicose veins

Infection

Malignancy

Estrogen therapy

Obesity

Prolonged surgery

Deficiencies of protein C, S, or antithrombin III

Factor V mutation

Prothrombin gene mutation

○ **T/F: Oral contraceptives should be stopped due to increased risk of DVT.**

False. Although no studies to date state a clinical benefit to stopping oral contraceptives, it is known that the hypercoagulable state lasts 4–6 weeks after birth control pills are stopped. One study gave a post op rate of DVT in those who used OCs as 0.96% compared to 0.5% to those who do not use OCs.

○ **What are the general recommendations of DVT prophylaxis?**

Low risk: encourage leg movement while in bed or provide a footboard for those not likely to ambulate, elastic stockings.

Moderate risk: same as for low risk, plus heparin 5,000 units subcutaneous tid with initial dose 2 hours prior to surgery. Low molecular weight heparin and or sequential pneumatic compression stockings can be employed prior to anesthesia induction.

High risk: same as for low risk and moderate risk plus heparin 5,000 units SC tid continued until patient is ambulatory, usually 1–2 days prior to discharge.

○ **What are the common causes of postoperative oliguria (inability to urinate)?**

Prerenal.

Most common cause of low urine output is hypovolemia.

External fluids loss i.e. hemorrhage, dehydration and diarrhea treat with fluids, Internal or third space loss, i.e., bowel obstruction, pancreatitis.

Congestive heart failure.

Renal—nephrotoxic medications can cause decreased urine output and if above prerenal causes are not corrected, can result in acute tubular necrosis.

Postrenal, i.e., prostatic hypertrophy, blocked Foley, stone in solitary kidney.

Most important is to assess the hydration of the patient, are they dry or in failure? Monitor hourly urine outputs via Foley.

○ **When dealing with outpatient surgical care, what are the diagnostic criteria for discharge?**

Stable vital signs

Return of protective reflexes including

Lacrimal duct involvement

Presence of ptosis

○ **What are the two purposes of abdominal drains?**

Provides for escape of infection/pus.

Removal of any fluids in the peritoneal cavity, i.e., bile, pancreatic juices in appropriate cases.

○ **When dealing with multisystem trauma, especially involving motor vehicular crashes, there is a 35% risk of this complication arising.**
What is it?

Fat embolization or fat embolism syndrome can result in hypoxia, confusion, petechiae, agitation, stupor, and tachycardia with progressive hypoxia.

This syndrome can occur on the second to fourth day following injury with diagnosis made using arterial PO_2 (usually less than 60), presence of fat emboli, fat globules in the urine and elevated free fatty acid levels.

Prevention by monitoring for risk factors, presence of a low circulating albumin and preventative treatment with albumin to maintain a circulating level of 3 gm per 100 ml.

Treatment consists of ventilatory support with endotracheal intubation and PEEP on volume cycled respirator.

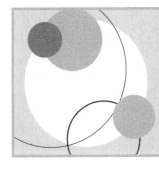

Bibliography

BOOKS/ARTICLES

Advanced Cardiac Life Support. Dallas, TX: American Heart Association, 2005.

Advanced Trauma Life Support. Chicago, IL: American College of Surgeons, 2004.

Anderson, J.E. Grant's Atlas of Anatomy (10th edn). Baltimore, MD: Lippincott Williams & Wilkins, 1999.

Auerbach, P.S. Management of Wilderness and Environmental Emergencies (3rd edn). St. Louis, MO: Mosby, 1995.

Beare, P.G. Adult Health Nursing (3rd edn). St. Louis, MO: Mosby, 1998.

Berkow, R. The Merck Manual (18th edn). Rahway: Merck Sharp & Dohme Research Laboratories, 2006.

Black, J.M. Medical-Surgical Nursing (7th edn). Philadelphia, PA: Saunders, 2005.

Braunwald, E., Fauci, A.S., Kasper, D.L. Harrison's Principles of Internal Medicine (15th edn). New York: McGraw-Hill, 2001.

Bryson, P.D. Comprehensive Review in Toxicology for Emergency Clinicians (3rd edn). Garland Publishing, 1996.

Dambro, M.R. Griffith's 5 Minute Clinical Consult (11th edn). Baltimore, MD: Lippincott Williams & Wilkins, 2003.

DeGowin, E.L. Bedside Diagnostic Examination (6th edn). New York: Macmillan, 1999.

Edwards, L. Dermatology in Emergency Care. London: Churchill Livingstone, 1997.

Fitzpatrick, T.B. Color Atlas and Synopsis of Clinical Dermatology (4th edn). New York: McGraw-Hill, 2000.

Frye, C. Frye's 2000 Nursing Bullets (3rd edn). Springhouse, PA: Springhouse Corp, 1994.

Gingrich, Margaret, M. Medical-Surgical Nursing (2nd edn). Springhouse, PA: Springhouse Corp, 2000.

Gunn, V.L. The Harriet Lane Handbook (16th edn). Philadelphia, PA: Saunders, 2002.

Harris, J.H. The Radiology of Emergency Medicine (4th edn). Baltimore, MD: Lippincott Williams & Wilkins, 1999.

Harwood-Nuss, A. The Clinical Practice of Emergency Medicine (3rd edn). Philadelphia: Lippincott Williams & Wilkin Company, 2001.

Healy, P. American Nursing Review, Questions and Answers for NCLEX RN (2nd edn). Springhouse, PA: Springhouse Corporation, 2001.

Holleran, R. Emergency and Flight Nursing Review (2nd edn). St. Louis, MO: Mosby, 1996.

Ignatavicius, D.D. Medical-Surgical Nursing (5th edn). Philadelphia, PA: Saunders 2006.

Kidd, P. Emergency Nursing. Springhouse, PA: Springhouse Corp, 1997.

Koenig, K. Emergency Medicine PreTest, Self-Assessment and Review. New York: McGraw-Hill, 2000.

Lester, B. The Acute Hand. Stamford, CT: Appleton & Lange, 1998.

Lewis, S.M. Medical-Surgical Nursing (6th edn). St. Louis, MO: Mosby, 2004.

Marriott, H.J.L. Practical Electrocardiography (10th edn). Baltimore, MD: Williams and Wilkins, 2000.

Medical-Surgical Nursing Certification (3rd edn). Baltimore, MD: Lippincott Williams & Wilkins, 2002.

Monahan, F.D. Phipps' Medical-Surgical Nursing: Foundations for Clinical Practice (8th edn). St. Louis, MO: Mosby, 2006.

Moore, K.L. Clinically Oriented Anatomy (4th edn). Baltimore, MD: Lippincott Williams & Wilkins, 2000.

Nettina, S.M. The Lippincott Manual of Nursing Practice (7th edn). Philadelphia: Lippincott Company, 2000.

Phipps, W.J., Cassmeyer, V.L., Sands, J.K. Medical Surgical Nursing: Concepts and Clinical Practice (5th edn). Elsevier Science Health Division, 1995.

Physicians' Desk Reference (57th edn). Oradell, NJ: Medical Economics Company, 2003.

Pillitteri, A. Maternal and Child Health Nursing: Care of the Childbearing and Childrearing Family (4th edn). Philadelphia: Lippincott Williams & Wilkin, 2002.

Plantz, S.H. Emergency Medicine: Pearls of Wisdom (6th edn). New York: McGraw-Hill, 2005.

Rosen, P. Emergency Medicine Concepts and Clinical Practice (5th edn). Elsevier Science Health Division, 2002.

Rudolph, A.M. Fundamentals of Pediatrics (3rd edn). New York: McGraw-Hill/Appleton & Lange, 2001.

Shives, L.R. Basic Concepts of Psychiatric-Mental Health Nursing (5th edn). Baltimore, MD: Lippincott Williams & Wilkins, 2001.

Simon, R.R. Emergency Orthopedics: The Extremities (5th edn). New York: McGraw-Hill, 2006.

Smeltzer, Suzanne Brunner and Suddarth's Textbook of Medical-Surgical Nursing (10th edn). Philadelphia: Lippincott Williams & Wilkins, 2004.

Stedman, T.L. Stedman's Medical Dictionary (27th edn). Baltimore, MD: Lippincott Williams & Wilkins, 2003.

Swearingen, Pamela, L. Manual of Medical-Surgical Nursing Care (5th edn). St. Louis, MO: Mosby, 2003.

The Hand Examination and Diagnosis (3rd edn). London: Churchill Livingstone, 1990.

The Hand Primary Care of Common Problems (2nd edn). London: Churchill Livingstone, 1990.

Tintinalli, J.E. Emergency Medicine: A Comprehensive Study Guide (6th edn). New York: McGraw-Hill, 2003.

Weinberg, S. Color Atlas of Pediatric Dermatology (3rd edn). New York: McGraw-Hill, 1997.

Weiner, H.L. Neurology for the House Officer (4th edn). Baltimore, MD: Lippincott Williams & Wilkins, 1989.

Whaley, L.F., Wong, D.L. Whaley & Wong's Essentials of Pediatric Nursing (7th edn). St. Louis, MO: Mosby Year Book, 2004.

Wilkins, E.W. Emergency Medicine (3rd edn). Baltimore, MD: Lippincott Williams & Wilkins, 1989.